Chronic Kidney Disease - Novel Insights into Pathophysiology and Treatment

Edited by Giovanni Palleschi and Valeria Rossi

Published in London, United Kingdom

Chronic Kidney Disease - Novel Insights into Pathophysiology and Treatment
http://dx.doi.org/10.5772/intechopen.1002113
Edited by Giovanni Palleschi and Valeria Rossi

Contributors
Ali Alkatheeri, Ana Paula Silva, Blerim Mujaj, Chanaka Jayasinghe, Daria Sergeevna Sadovskaya, Eduarda Carias, Giovanni Palleschi, Henriques Borges, Hermínio Carrasqueira, José Soares, Kogila Supramanian, Mahendran Sekar, Mohd. Aslam, Mohd. Hatif, Nevil Rajakaruna, Nor Safwan Hadi Nor Afendi, Randah Dahlan, Rita Afonso, Roberto Calças Marques, Stellor Nlandu Khodo, Thushara Hewageegana, Venera Berisha-Muharremi

First published in London, United Kingdom, 2024 by IntechOpen
IntechOpen is the global imprint of INTECHOPEN LIMITED, registered in England and Wales, registration number: 11086078, 167-169 Great Portland Street, London, W1W 5PF, United Kingdom

British Library Cataloguing-in-Publication Data
A catalogue record for this book is available from the British Library

Additional hard and PDF copies can be obtained from orders@intechopen.com

Chronic Kidney Disease - Novel Insights into Pathophysiology and Treatment
Edited by Giovanni Palleschi and Valeria Rossi
p. cm.
Print ISBN 978-0-85466-653-9
Online ISBN 978-0-85466-652-2
eBook (PDF) ISBN 978-0-85466-654-6

For EU product safety concerns:
IN TECH d.o.o., Prolaz Marije Krucifikse Kozulić 3, 51000 Rijeka, Croatia,
info@intechopen.com or visit our website at intechopen.com.

Meet the editors

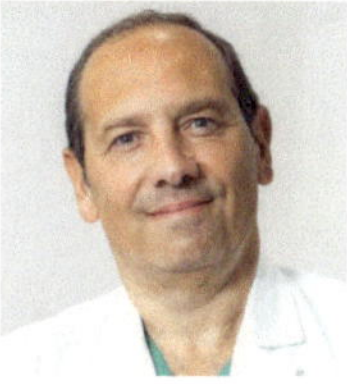

Giovanni Palleschi (MD, Ph.D.) graduated in 1997 and specialized in urology in 2002 at Sapienza University of Rome. In 2002 he won a prize for research on anatomo-clinical correlations of urinary disorders in patients with multiple sclerosis, and in 2011 he achieved a physician doctorate in human anatomy, dermatology, and plastic surgery. He has been a member of the Scientific Committees of the Italian Society of Urology, the Italian Society of Urodynamics, and the European Association of Urology. He participated as a co-investigator in numerous clinical trials. He is the author of 70 publications edited on PubMed and scientific books. He participated in academic teaching activities at the Sapienza University of Rome. At present, he is a consultant urologist for the Nefrocenter Group (Italy).

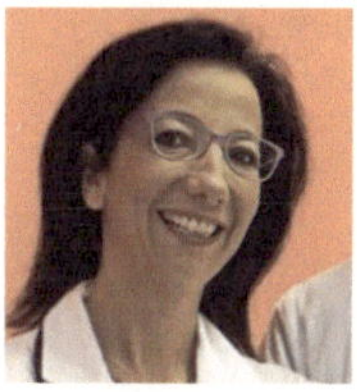

Valeria Rossi, MD, graduated in 2000 from Sapienza University of Rome and specialized in nephrology in 2005 at Tor Vergata University of Rome. She has great experience as a clinical nephrologist in public healthcare hospitals, then as chief of hemodialysis centers since 2009, and is an expert on surgical management of vascular accesses for hemodialysis. She has published various manuscripts on diabetic nephropathy and hemodialysis techniques and has participated as co-editor of scientific books. At present, she is the chief of the Hemodialysis Center of Frascati (Rome) of the Nefrocenter Group (Italy).

Contents

Preface

Chronic kidney disease (CKD) is a pathological condition with high prevalence in the world, and it is responsible for a significant socioeconomic burden. A large number of patients suffer from this chronic disorder as a complication of systemic diseases, mainly blood hypertension and diabetes. Chronic kidney disease causes various pathophysiological consequences, inducing anemia, disorders of calcium and phosphorus metabolism, and secondary immunodeficiency. The most important clinical aspect is that CKD is strongly associated with an increased cardiovascular risk and represents one of the main pathological conditions with an increased risk of death. These risks are particularly represented in patients undergoing replacement therapy (extracorporeal hemodialysis and peritoneal dialysis) due to additional possible complications related to the type of treatment.

Lifestyle changes, especially regarding dietetic aspects, smoke abuse, and pollution, have significantly contributed to a worrying incidence of dysmetabolic, cardiovascular, and oncologic pathologies that are also often responsible for or associated with CKD. Therefore the prevalence and incidence of CKD are both continuously increasing at this time, and medical assistance for patients will surely represent a challenge in the next years. Compared to the past, therapeutic options to manage this condition have greatly improved. Furthermore, progress in kidney transplant provides better outcomes, with improved survival rates and lower incidence of severe complications, even if the organ supply is still inadequate to the demand. Considering these aspects, the incoming years are going to present new challenges for patients suffering from CKD, and healthcare systems have the responsibility to offer the best medical assistance. For this reason, clinical research has a pivotal role in this field and has provided new insights into the pathophysiology and treatment of CKD.

In this book, some of the most important topics regarding new knowledge about CKD are reported. After an introductory section that explains the aim of the project and summarizes the most significant epidemiological and clinical aspects of CKD, the subsequent chapters explore current important themes related to pathogenetic mechanisms and therapeutic approaches, with an emphasis on quality of life. Considering pathophysiologic aspects, the role of the epithelial TGF-β/β-catenin axis in proximal tubule response to CKD is reported. The following chapter is dedicated to CKD of unknown origin in Sri Lanka, with new insights into etiopathogenetic, clinical, and histologic data and providing a revision of the current literature. The subsequent chapters are focused on the nutritional aspects of CKD. The first one is dedicated to the important role of diet in this pathological condition. Dietary requirements and restrictions for patients suffering from CKD play a critical role in improving well-being and quality of life, contributing to optimized outcomes of treatment and preventing severe complications. The following chapter describes the pathophysiological mechanisms involved in the determination of kidney damage by adipose tissue, which represents a risk factor for CKD. Then, the role played by resistin in diabetic patients with CKD and its connections with nutritional status and cardiovascular outcomes is discussed in the next chapter. The book continues with a section dedicated to therapeutic aspects for patients suffering from CKD. One important chapter is focused on renoprotective strategies. Nowadays a multimodal approach to prevent kidney damage and to preserve residual renal function during CKD is recommended, and it includes dietary suggestions and the use of renoprotective drugs, some of which have been recently developed and introduced in clinical practice also for late stages of renal failure. Among drugs that are very important in the late stages of CKD and in patients suffering from end-stage renal disease who are under replacement therapy, potassium binders are the most important because they prevent a severe and potentially fatal complication: hyperkaliemia. New molecules capable of binding potassium are today available in the market for clinical application and are presented and discussed in the final chapter.

It is our honor and pleasure to thank all the contributors to this book for their efforts and their excellent work.

Giovanni Palleschi and Valeria Rossi
Nefrocenter Hemodialysis Center,
Medica San Carlo,
Frascati (Rome), Italy

Section 1

Overview, Etiology and Pathophysiology

Chapter 1

Introductory Chapter: Chronic Kidney Disease – Introductive Overview and Current Issues

Giovanni Palleschi

1. Introduction

Chronic kidney disease (CKD) is reported as a "kidney damage for ≥3 months, as defined by structural or functional abnormalities of the kidney, with or without decreased GFR" [1]. Chronic kidney disease has been classified into five different stages based on disease severity from mild condition to the end-stage renal disease (ESRD), which represents a status of complete renal failure and requires replacement therapy (dialysis or kidney transplantation) [2]. Chronic kidney disease may be the consequence of many pathologic conditions from genetic disorders to malformative alterations, inflammatory, degenerative, immunologic, metabolic, toxic, and oncologic pathologies. However, despite the numerous and various etiopathogenetic factors that can lead to CKD, a large part of patients suffering from this disorder are affected by blood hypertension and diabetes, which are two of the most prevalent pathologic conditions in the world. Lifestyle changes, especially regarding dietetic aspects, smoke abuse, and pollution, have hardly increase the risk to develop dysmetabolic, cardiovascular, and oncologic pathologies that are also often responsible for CKD. As a consequence, the prevalence and incidence of CKD are continuously increasing during the time and medical assistance for patients will become a challenge in the next years. New strategies for disease prevention to improve therapeutical options that can delay its progression, and new perspectives that could replace the invasive methods to treat ESRD are warranted to improve patients' quality of life, wellness of population, and to provide a favorable impact on public healthcare systems, being in most countries a significant economic burden to manage CKD patients and substantial inequity for them in access to medical services.

2. Epidemiologic and socio-economic aspects

Epidemiologic aspects of CKD are important to understand how much this pathologic condition could have a negative socio-economic impact. Chronic kidney disease is highly represented in the general population, accounting more than 800 million individuals [3]. Furthermore, this disorder has presented a significant increase of incidence and prevalence in the last 10 years, and it is one of the most frequent causes of death [4]. Recent review studies, including rigorous metanalysis of epidemiological investigations performed on large populations, report a prevalence of CKD varying from 10.6 to 13.4% [5]. One of the most important characteristics of CKD, under a social point of view, is that patients affected by this condition have an increased risk to death that has been estimated from one to five times higher than general population. This specific risk increases with disease severity, being the most in subjects with renal failure undergoing dialysis [5]. Patients suffering from CKD need continuous medical assistance since early stages of condition to advanced ones. General clinical status worsens with progression of CKD requiring laboratory tests to assess kidney function, imaging of urinary tract, and cardiovascular assessment. Nutritional restrictions, medical pharmacological treatment, or invasive therapies (i.e., peritoneal or extracorporeal hemodialysis) are differently provided basing on the CKD stage. As a consequence, patients' quality of life (QoL) proportionally decreases either due to clinical conditions related to the renal disorder or also due to the need of recurrent diagnostic and therapeutic interventions. Most important studies on patients with CKD show that QoL falls with disease progression, especially in patients with significant comorbidities such as diabetes, and that it is particularly compromised in those undergoing dialysis [6]. The same studies assess that renal transplantation has the most favorable impact on QoL of CKD patients if compared with all the other treatments available for ESRD because it provides the most valuable functional ability [7]. During the last years, the incidence and prevalence increase of CKD have presented the same epidemiological trend shown by blood hypertension and diabetes, which have been identified as the main responsible for CKD [8]. Blood hypertension still represents the principal cardiovascular risk factor [8], and therefore, CKD significantly worsens the cardiovascular risk of individuals, independently from sex and age, but proportionally to stage disorder. Large epidemiological surveys show that CKD can be considered one of the most important causes of death throughout the world [8]. There is still somewhat controversy about epidemiological findings of CKD because the studies during the time have used different methods for its definition and classification [9]. However, there is a common scientific agreement that the burden of CKD is considerable, taking into account also direct and indirect costs of population needing diagnostic assessments, medical treatments, and replacement therapy (hemodialysis, peritoneal dialysis, and renal transplantation), whose number has been estimated approximately between 4902 and 7083 million people [10]. All these data and considerations should enforce the need of a general awareness about this pathologic condition and the possible future evolution in terms of incidence, prevalence, impact on Qol, and economic burden, especially considering aging of population, which directly correlates to functional kidney impairment. Some studies have provided data about the estimation of the increase of nephropathic population in the next years. In European countries, a number of people with CKD over 100 million are expected [10]. This will surely induce the governments, sanitary systems, and social services to develop more prevention strategies to reduce the impact of CKD on the world population and will prompt medical research to improve nephroprotective measures and therapeutic options, aiming to limit the number of patients who will need replacement therapies.

3. Current issues of chronic kidney disease

After the beginning of the new century, we have assisted to significant changes under epidemiological point of view regarding health status [11]. World population is continuously aging and chronic pathologic conditions are getting even more prevalent proportionally to this phenomenon. Particularly, a consistent decrease of diseases than can be transmitted has been associated with a severe increase of risk factors of chronic non-transmissible pathologies [12]. In this scenario, CKD has presented, as above mentioned, a significant increase of incidence and prevalence, and the identification of risk factors and their treatment is the most important action to adopt aiming to reduce the CKD burden. Various levels of intervention can be applied to reach this goal. Nutrition campaigns, that today can be delivered also by social media, to reduce dysmetabolic syndromes (dyslipidemia, diabetes), obesity, and smoking (which are strongly associated to cardiovascular risk) should be supported, and educational strategies should be developed since the first years of school to limit also the onset of the same disorders in the pediatrics and adolescents [13]. All these strategies have the goal to reduce the number of people suffering from chronic diseases, including CKD, and can contribute to lower the socio-economic impact of this condition on public healthcare. The strongest effort regarding prevention should be focused on diabetes and blood hypertension, which result to be the principal risk factors for CKD in all countries. Unfortunately, promotion of these preventive actions is difficult to achieve with the same efficacy in all the countries being these initiatives directly under the control of different governments. However, various experiences with campaigns of screening and prevention performed in different countries on adult and young people (middle school) have shown to be feasible and to increase awareness of population, among the public and policymakers [14–16]. Very important studies confirm that screening and prevention programs can prevent CKD and that in those countries that adopted and implemented management strategies the incidence of ESRD has been reduced [17]. These experiences should convince about the utility of prevention programs to limit the impact on the population of chronic pathologic conditions, requiring in the future more economic investments. In fact, early detection of chronic conditions is often based on the identification of biological markers as predictors of disease and that have high costs if widely investigated on large populations. One of the most important aspects that can prompt the governments and public healthcare systems to face the clinical and socio-economic impact of CKD is represented by the costs that this chronic disease requires for diagnosis and treatment of patients. Some studies report that almost 70–80% of sanitary resources of public healthcare are spent to manage chronic diseases [17]. Specific data from European countries estimate annual costs at about 700 billion euro that are comprehensive of direct costs (for diagnostic and therapeutic procedures) but mostly of the indirect ones (absence from work, nutritional support, and psychological care) [18]. In particular, in patients for CKD, it has been shown that these costs are directly correlated with disease progression reaching about 52,000 euros/patient per year in those undergoing hemodialysis. Therefore, prevention strategies and rigorous therapeutic approach should be adopted to strongly reduce the rate of patients undergoing replacement therapies, offering people with CKD better QoL and hardly reducing costs for public healthcare. Recent improvements on pathophysiology of CKD have contributed to develop better therapeutic options to manage conservative treatment. In addition to the well-known and commonly used pharmacologic treatments (as ACE inhibitors and angiotensin receptor antagonists or sartans) [19], new drugs are today available with renoprotective effects. Glucagon-like peptide-1 receptor agonists, dipeptidyl peptidase-4 inhibitors, and sodium-glucose cotransporter 2 inhibitors represent a new frontier as glucose-lowering agents for diabetic CKD, having a significant renoprotective effect that can slow the disease progression and delay the need of replacement therapy [20, 21]. Additionally, in specific disorders, such as in Lupus Nephritis, biological agents (belimumab, obinutuzumab, anifrolumab, et al.) have shown to provide renoprotective effects by modulating self-antigens or by dual immunosuppressive and antiproteinuric effects (voclosporin) [22]. Furthermore, it has been shown that in lupus nephritis sodium-glucose cotransporter 2 inhibitors alleviate podocyte damage, therefore, producing renoprotective effects [23]. Some interesting perspectives are also under investigation for patients suffering from polycystic kidney disease. In fact, new randomized clinical trials are going to assess the efficacy of new molecules acting on specific pathophysiological pathways and sphingolipids, and preliminary data suggest that in the future, the prognosis of these patients could improve [24]. These evidences induce to consider that in the future, the chance to lower the incidence and prevalence at least of ESRD can be considered realistic, and the use of these new pharmacologic options should theoretically have a lower economic impact if compared with that associated with replacement treatments. The efforts of governments and health systems should be focused on screening, prevention, health education, and research in order to reduce as much as possible the epidemiological trend toward growth of the population affected by CKD. On the other side, scientific societies have the responsibility to implement research in this field and disseminate knowledge on recent therapeutic advances to protect renal function. Although it is still far from real-life application, a very promising solution will probably income in the next 10 years for patients with ESRD needing replacement treatment and could be represented by the bionic kidney. This device is under pre-clinical assessment and it consists of an implantable system and a bioreactor. The bionic kidney is capable of functioning as a filter for the blood and to maintain the plasmatic homeostasis, but at the moment research is still far from clinical applications in humans, while preliminary data on animals have already published [25]. At the present, kidney transplant still represents the best solution for patients with renal failure. The number of kidney transplanted patients in the world has reported over 25,000 in 2022, and this number is expected to be larger from data under revision of 2023 considering the increasing number of donor nephrectomies (from living kidney donors) [26]. New surgical devices, especially robot-assisted procedures, have contributed to improve patients' compliance versus this type of surgery because less invasive. Furthermore, a better awareness of population about the need of kidney donation has hardly contributed to relief many patients from dialysis. The hope is that in the next years, all the efforts to reduce CKD incidence will help also to reduce the request of renal transplants, lowering the number of single-kidney individuals due to a donor nephrectomy.

4. Conclusion

Epidemiological and socio-economic data estimate a worrying growth of the population affected by CKD in the world, with consequent increase of mortality risk associated with this pathology, reduction of quality of life, and a significant economic impact on healthcare systems. Various scientific evidences show that this trend could be slowed down by screening and prevention programs and by the use of new therapeutic resources today available to protect kidney function. More than being a nephrological problem, nephroprotection has become a public health issue as the etiopathogenetic factors associated with it are represented by the most widespread chronic diseases, such as diabetes and hypertension, which are often related to malnutrition, especially overweight and obesity. For this reason, all institutions should be involved in programs intended to reduce the impact of CKD, including schools, responsible for very important educational aspects.

Author details

Giovanni Palleschi
Nefrocenter, Medica San Carlo, Frascati, Rome, Italy

*Address all correspondence to: giovanni.palleschi@santagostino.it

References

[1] K/DOQI. Clinical practice guidelines for chronic kidney disease. American Journal of Kidney Diseases. 2002;**39**:S1

[2] Ammirati R. Chronic kidney disease. Revista da Associação Médica Brasileira (1992). 2020;**66**(Suppl. 1):s03-s09. DOI: 10.1590/1806-9282.66.S1.3

[3] Kovesdy CP. Epidemiology of chronic kidney disease: An update 2022. Kidney International Supplements. 2002;**12**(1):7-11

[4] Hill NR, Fatoba ST, Oke JL, et al. Global prevalence of chronic kidney disease - A systematic review and meta-analysis. PLoS One. 2016;**11**:1-18

[5] Rhee CM, Kovesdy CP. Epidemiology: Spotlight on CKD deaths-increasing mortality worldwide. Nature Reviews. Nephrology. 2015;**11**:199

[6] Webster AC, Nagler EV, Morton RL, Masson P. Chronic kidney disease. Lancet. 2017;**389**(10075):1238-1252

[7] Parsons DS, Harris DC. A review of quality of life in chronic renal failure. PharmacoEconomics. 1997;**12**(2 Pt. 1): 140-160

[8] Centers for Disease Control and Prevention Chronic Kidney Disease (CKD) Surveillance System. 2021. Available from: https://nccd.cdc.gov/ckd/default.aspx [Accessed: September 30, 2021]

[9] Mills KT et al. A systematic analysis of worldwide population-based data on global burden of chronic kidney disease in 2010. Kidney International. Nov 2015;**88**(5):950-957

[10] Ji-Cheng LV, Zhang L-X. Prevalence and disease burden of chronic kidney disease. Advances in Experimental Medicine and Biology. 2019;**1165**:3-15

[11] Rothenberg R, Lentzner HR, Parker RA. Population aging patterns: The expansion of mortality. Journal of Gerontology. 1991;**46**(2):S66-S70. DOI: 10.1093/geronj/46.2.s66

[12] Chen X, Wang W, Qin Y, Zou J, Yu H. Global epidemiology of human infections with variant influenza viruses: 1959-2021: A descriptive study. Clinical Infectious Diseases. 2022;**75**(8):1315-1323. DOI: 10.1093/cid/ciac168

[13] Rogers A, Wilkinson S, Downie O, Truby H. Communication of nutrition information by influencers on social media: A scoping review. Health Promotion Journal of Australia. 2022;**33**(3):657-676. DOI: 10.1002/hpja.563. Epub 2022 Jan 4

[14] Mensah GA, Fuster V, Murray CJL, Roth GA. Global burden of cardiovascular diseases and risks collaborators. Global burden of cardiovascular diseases and risk, 1990-2022. Journal of the American College of Cardiology. 2023;**82**(25):2350-2473. DOI: 10.1016/j.jacc.2023.11.007

[15] Bovet P, Hirsiger P, Emery F, De Bernardini J, Rossier C, Trebeljahr J, et al. Impact and cost of a 2-week community based screening and awarness program for diabetes and cardiovascular risk in a Swiss canton. Diabetes, Metabolic Syndrome and Obesity. 2011;**4**:213-223. DOI: 10.2147/DMSO.S20649. Epub 2011 Jun 16

[16] Willi SM, Hirst K, Jago R, Buse J, Kaufman F, El Ghormli L, et al. Cardiovascular risk factors in ulti-ethnic middle school students: The

healthy primary prevention trial. Pediatric Obesity. 2012;**7**(3):230-239. DOI: 10.1111/j.2047-6310.2011.00042.x. Epub 2012 Mar 28

[17] Jha V, Garcia-Garcia G, Iseki K, Li Z, Naicker S, Plattner B, et al. Chronic kidney disease: Global dimension and perspectives. Lancet. 2013;**382**(9888):260-272. DOI: 10.1016/S0140-6736(13)60687-X. Epub 2013 May 31

[18] Kainz A, Hronsky M, Stel VS, Jager KJ, Geroldinger A, Dunkler D, et al. Prediction of prevalence of chronic kidney disease in diabetic patients in countries of the European Union up to 2025. Nephrology, Dialysis, Transplantation. 2015;**30**(Suppl. 4):iv113-iv118. DOI: 10.1093/ndt/gfv073

[19] Hsu FY, Lin FJ, Ou HT, Huang SH, Wang CC. Renoprotective effect of angiotensine converting enzyme inhibitors and angiotensin II receptor blockers in diabetic patients with proteinuria. Kidney & Blood Pressure Research. 2017;**42**(2):358-368. DOI: 10.1159/000477946. Epub 2017 Jun 15

[20] Sloan LA. Review of glucagon like peptide-1 receptor antagonist for the treatment of type 2 diabetes mellitus in patients with chronic kidney disease and their renal effects. Journal of Diabetes. 2019;**11**(12):938-948. DOI: 10.1111/1753-0407.12969. Epub 2019 Aug 14

[21] Heerspink HJL, Kosiborod M, Inzucchi SE, Cherney DZI. Renoprotective effects of sodium-glucose cotransporter-2 inhibitors. Kidney International. 2018;**94**(1):26-39. DOI: 10.1016/j.kint.2017.12.027. Epub 2018 May 5

[22] Kale A, Lech M, Anders HJ, Gaikwad AB. BioDrugs. 2023;**37**(4):463-475. DOI: 10.1007/s40259-023-00597-3. Epub 2023 Apr 24

[23] Zhao XY, Li SS, He YX, Yan LJ, Lv F, Liang QM, et al. SGLT2 inhibitors alleviate podocyte damage in luous nephritis by decreasing inflammation and enhancing autophagy. Annals of the Rheumatic Diseases. 2023;**82**(10):1328-1340. DOI: 10.1136/ard-2023-224242. Epub 2023 Jul 24

[24] Capuanno I, Buonanno P, Riccio E, Amicone M, Pisani A. Therapeutic advances in ADPKD: The future awaits. Journal of Nephrology. 2022;**35**(2):397-415. DOI: 10.1007/s40620-021-01062-6. Epub 2021 May 19

[25] Bonomini V. Artificial Cells, Blood Substitutes, and Immobilization Biotechnology. 2003;**31**(2):105-110

[26] Artiles A et al. Kidney transplant outcomes in elderly population: A systematic review and meta-analysis. European Urology Open Science. Kidney International. Nov 2015;**88**(5):950-957. DOI: 10.1038/ki.2015.230. Epub 2015 Jul 29

Chapter 2

Chronic Kidney Disease: Etiology, Pathophysiology, and Management Strategies to Increase Quality of Life

Kogila Supramanian, Mahendran Sekar and Nor Safwan Hadi Nor Afendi

Abstract

Chronic kidney disease (CKD) refers to a variety of pathophysiologic conditions linked to poor kidney function and persistent reduction in glomerular filtration rate. According to the National Kidney Foundation's guidelines, CKD can be classified based on the amount of glomerular filtration rate. There are numerous etiologies for the occurrence of CKD. Various medications used to treat CKD will include slowing the progression, which is medical treatment, as well as employing natural products. Many strategies can be used to improve the quality of life of a CKD patient. This book chapter will further discuss etiology, pathophysiology, clinical manifestation, investigation, and management of patients in renal replacement therapy and also usage of medication to increase the quality of life.

Keywords: chronic kidney disease, glomerular filtration rate, quality of life, medical treatment, severity of illness

1. Introduction

1.1 Chronic kidney disease (CKD)

CKD, or known as chronic renal failure (CRF), describes all degrees of decreased kidney function, ranging from damaged-at-risk to mild, moderate, and severe chronic kidney failure [1]. A patient can be confirmed as CKD when the estimated glomerular filtration rate (eGFR) becomes less than 60 ml/min per 1.73 square meters, persisting for 3 months or more. It is a progressive loss of kidney function that eventually necessitates renal replacement therapy (dialysis or transplantation). This activity reviews the etiology, evaluation, and management of chronic kidney disease and emphasizes the roles of the interprofessional team in the care of chronic kidney disease patients. Pathologic abnormalities in urinary sediment, abnormalities in urinary albumin excretion rates, or increased urinary albumin excretion rates are all examples of kidney damage. The Kidney Disease Improving Global Outcome (KDIGO) has classified details about the causes of CKD, and it is classified into six categories based on eGFR, as stated in **Table 1**. Stage 3 has been classified into 3a and 3b in the year of 2012 according to the eGFR and clinical manifestation. It also includes albuminuria staging (A1, A2, and A3), with each stage of CKD subcategorized based on the urinary albumin-creatinine ratio in (mg/gm) or (mg/mmol) in an early morning "spot" urine sample as in **Table 2** [2]. The Kidney Disease Outcome Quality Initiative (KDOQI) provides a guideline to classify CKD developed in 1997 that was revised in 2012. Albuminuria has been added as a predictor outcome as well [3].

1.2 Etiology of CKD

The causes of CKD vary globally, and the following are the most common primary diseases that cause CKD and, ultimately, end-stage renal disease (ESRD) has been demonstrated in **Figure 1**.

i. *Diabetes mellitus type 2*

The kidney's filtering units are filled with tiny blood vessels. High blood sugar levels can cause these vessels to narrow and clog over time. When there is insufficient blood, the kidneys suffer damage, and albumin passes through these filters and ends up in the urine, where it should not be.

ii. *Diabetes mellitus type 1*

About 30% of Type 1 (juvenile-onset) diabetes patients and 10 to 40% of Type 2 (adult-onset) diabetes patients will eventually develop kidney failure.

Stage	Description	GFR (mL/min/1.73m^2)
1	Kidney damage with normal or high GFR	>90
2	Mild decrease in GFR	60–89
3a	Mild-to-moderate decrease in GFR	45–59
3b	Moderate to deVere decrease in GFR	30–44
4	Severely decrease GFR	15–29
5	Kidney failure	<15 or dialysis

Table 1.
Classification of CKD by GFR (KDIGO 2012).

Category	Albumin excretion rate (mg/24 h)	Albumin: creatinine ratio (mg/mmol)	Terms
A1	<30	<3	Normal to mildly increased
A2	30–300	3–30	Moderately increased
A3	>300	>30	Severely increased

Table 2.
Albuminuria categories in CKD (KDIGO 2012).

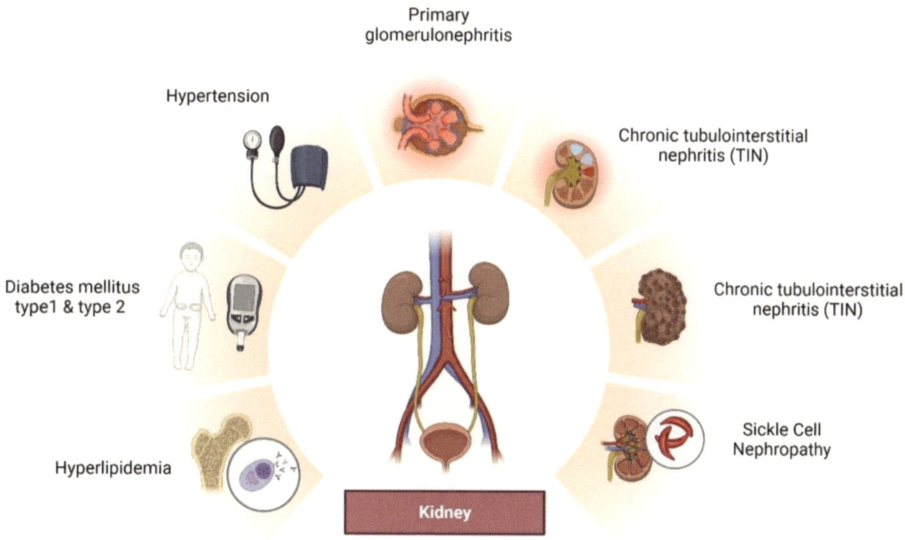

Figure 1.
Examples of diseases related to chronic kidney disease (CKD).

iii. *Hypertension*

High blood pressure can constrict and narrow blood vessels, causing them to become damaged and weak throughout the body, including the kidneys. Blood flow is reduced due to the narrowing. If the blood vessels in your kidneys are damaged, they may no longer function properly. When this occurs, kidneys are unable to remove all waste and excess fluid from body. Extra fluid in the blood vessels can raise blood pressure even higher, starting a dangerous cycle that can lead to kidney failure.

iv. *Primary glomerulonephritis*

Chronic inflammation of glomerulus causes long-term kidney damage and decline in function. Chronic kidney disease is defined as kidney damage or decreased function lasting 3 months or longer. Chronic kidney disease can progress to end-stage kidney disease, requiring dialysis or a kidney transplant.

v. *Chronic tubulointerstitial nephritis (TIN)*

GFR is reduced in acute TIN due to interstitial edema, lymphocyte and plasma cell infiltration, and poor tubular function. The decrease in GFR in chronic TIN is caused by fibrosis of the interstitium rather than edema. If prolonged, acute interstitial inflammatory reactions can lead to accumulation of extracellular matrix that causes irreversible impairment of renal function with interstitial fibrosis and tubular atrophy.

vi. *Hereditary or Cystic Disease*

Cystic kidney disease (CKD) refers to a group of conditions that result in the formation of cysts (fluid-filled sacs) in or around the kidneys. Kidney cysts can obstruct the kidneys' ability to filter water and waste from your blood. Kidney failure can result from cystic kidney disease.

vii. *Plasma Cell Dyscariasis or Neoplasm*

Renal disease in myeloma is typically characterized by renal insufficiency and proteinuria. Patients with myeloma may occasionally present with renal tubular dysfunction, including acidification and concentration defects and, in rare cases, the Fanconi syndrome.

viii. *Sickle Cell Nephropathy*

Sickle cell disease causes damage to multiple structures within the kidney.
Chronic anemia's hemodynamic changes, renal hypoxia caused by recurrent vaso-occlusion, and hemolysis-related endothelial dysfunction can all lead to functional and structural changes that can progress to CKD.

1.3 Pathophysiology of CKD

The rate of renal blood flow, which is approximately 400 ml/100 g of tissue per minute, is significantly higher than that observed in other well-perfused vascular beds such as the heart, liver, and brain. When there are any harmful circulating agents or substances, there is a higher chance that renal tissue might be exposed to them [4]. In contrast to other capillary beds, glomerular filtration is dependent on relatively high intra- and trans-glomerular pressure, even under physiological settings, which makes glomerular capillaries prone to hemodynamic damage. The details of the disease process are shown in **Figure 2**.

The major contributors to the progression of chronic kidney disease could be hypertension and hyperfiltration. Negatively charged molecules in the glomerular filtration membrane act as a barrier, slowing anionic macromolecules. When this electrostatic barrier is breached, as occurs in many types of glomerular damage,

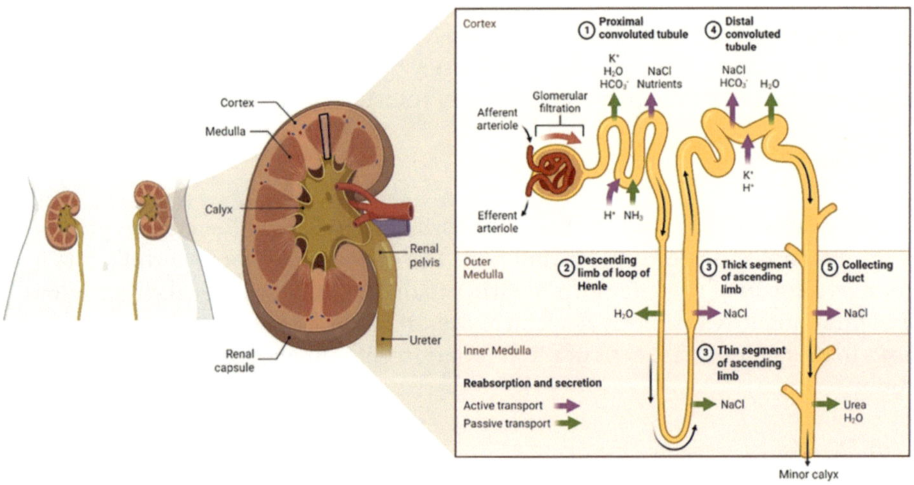

Figure 2.
Diagrammatic representation of the glomerulus function in the process of reabsorption and secretion.

plasma protein gains access to the glomerular filtrate. The sequential organization of the nephron's microvasculature and the downstream position of the tubule with respect to the glomeruli not only maintains the glomerulo-tubular balance but also allows glomerular injury to spread to the tubulointerstitial compartment in disease, exposing tubular epithelial cells to abnormal ultrafiltrate [5]. Due to the peritubular vasculature underpins the glomerular circulation, some mediators of the glomerular inflammatory response may overflow into the peritubular circulation, contributing to the interstitial inflammatory responses commonly observed in glomerular illness. Tubulointerstitial injury and tissue remodeling will occur due to decrease in preglomerular or glomerular perfusion [6]. Therefore, the concept of the nephron as a functional unit relates not only to renal physiology but also to renal disease pathology. There are some main reasons that kidney can go into impairment such as immunologic reaction, tissue hypoxia, and ischemia, exogenic agents as drugs, endogenous substance as glucose or paraproteins, and hereditary [7].

1.4 Stages of CKD

CKD can be divided into five stages and six categories that range from 1 to 5. The determination of CKD with stages is done by blood investigation known as estimated glomerular filtration rate (eGFR). Stage 1 kidney disease has an estimated glomerular filtration of 90 or higher with a progressive kidney involvement of more than 3 months. The estimated glomerular filtration rate is an absolute indicator of kidneys function in the filtration of excess fluid from blood [8]. At every stage of CKD, the kidneys function progressively deteriorates and requires different treatment to slow down the damage to kidney that will keep them functioning as long as possible. A patient with renal failure will need to go on renal replacement therapy such as hemodialysis, peritoneal dialysis, or renal transplant to sustain life [9].

1.4.1 CKD stage 1

Stage 1 CKD is considered mild, and no significant clinical manifestation exists to address it. GFR is 90 mls/min. This stage is considered mild. It may have proteinuria, whereby there is leakage of protein in the urine allowed by glomeruli. Sometimes, changes can be noticed through ultrasound or microalbumin in the urine. Many times, patients may complain that they have foamy urine that is caused by excessive amounts of urine albumin.

To reduce the progression of kidney disease, it is advisable to monitor patients' blood pressure to be in health range under 120/80 mmHG. Also, it is important to control salt intake less than 2300 milligrams (mg) per day. There are also patients having difficulty in identifying hidden salt. If patients are known case of diabetes, they should have good control of their glucose [10].

1.4.2 CKD stage 2

The damage is still considered mild, yet the kidneys will be functioning to the optimum level with 20–40% normal function. GFR will 60-89 ml/min. The symptoms still remain as foamy urine.

A recommended lifestyle modification will include losing weight and considering a healthy diet. To delay the progress of CKD stage 2, a few conservative managements are recommended. For obese patients, it is recommended for them to lose weight through exercise. Quitting smoking can help lower blood pressure and reduce stress on the kidneys. Encouraging the patient to get enough sleep and manage stress will influence blood pressure as well. For diabetic patients, it is recommended to consume medication such as angiotensin-converting enzyme (ACE) inhibitors, angiotensin II receptor blockers (ARBs), sodium-glucose cotransporter 2 (SGLT2) inhibitors, or Kerendia which can slow down the progress of CKD.

1.4.3 CKD stage 3

At this stage, the patient will have symptoms that indicate enough damage to start producing symptoms. This happens when 15% of the function of normal kidney remains is attained. Stage 3 can be categorized into 3a and 3b. Stage 3a is kidney function having mild-to-moderate function loss with GFR 45–59 mL/min, whereas 3b is moderate-to-severe loss of kidney function with GFR 30–44 mL/min. At this point, a CKD patient may have developed anemia and renal osteodystrophy [11].

Clinical manifestations of stage 3a CKD may include:

- Polyuria or some patients may experience oliguria
- Fatigue and tiredness
- Dry or itchy skin
- Nausea
- Los of appetite
- Unintended weight loss

Clinical manifestations for CKD stage 3b may include:

- Unable to focus
- Muscle aches and cramping especially lower limbs
- Shortness of breath
- Peripheral edema (swelling in the arms, legs, hands, or feet)
- Peripheral neuropathy (numbness and tingling sensation in the hands and feet)

At this stage, the patient will be prescribed statin drugs to reduce cholesterol; administration of a diuretic will promote urination, reduce blood pressure, and reduce peripheral edema. For mineral bone disease, it is advisable to take calcium and vitamin D supplements. Anemia can be managed with iron supplements.

1.4.4 CKD stage 4

At this stage, kidneys have been impaired, moderate to severe with eGFR 15-29 mL/min. The complication of disease markedly increases like anemia, high blood pressure, bone disease, and metabolic acidosis. Also, there will be hyperkalemia and hyperphosphatemia that leads to cardiac dysrhythmia. Patients may experience persistent lower back pain, insomnia, ammonia breath smell, and microscopic or gross hematuria. At this stage, there is a need for treatment, and it includes dietary adjustment that the patients need for protein restriction. Low phosphate diet and low potassium diet will minimize the complication of electrolyte imbalance. Nephrotoxic drugs such as nonsteroidal anti-inflammatory drugs (NSAIDs), cephalosporins, statins, insulin, and proton pump inhibitors should be avoided. Low hemoglobin level can be treated using erythropoiesis-stimulating agents (ESAs). Although the treatment for CKD stage 4 uses medication to control symptoms, this medication itself can damage the kidney as well.

1.4.5 CKD stage 5

Stage 5 of CKD is the most alarming stage where the patient experiences kidney failure with eGFR<15 mls/min. The kidney function at this stage GFR drops to less than 15 mL/min, and if only 10% of the remaining kidney is there, this is considered as End-Stage Renal Disease (ESRD). Stage 5 is associated with uremia, whereby the waste product accumulates in the blood [12]. The patient will experience dyspnea, pruritus, chest pain, nausea and vomiting, restless leg syndrome, abnormal bruises, hiccups, seizure, and coma. At this stage, the treatment will include renal replacement therapy that is dialysis, either hemodialysis or peritoneal dialysis or kidney transplant.

System	Complication
Central nervous system	Difficulty concentrating, mood swing, seizure, depression, uremic encephalopathy, and coma.
Circulatory blood	Anemia, fluid and electrolyte imbalance, edema, metabolic acidosis, hyperkalemia, hyperphosphatemia, hypocalcemia, and bleeding tendency.
Cardiovascular system	Hypertension, cardiac dysrhythmia, left ventricular hypertrophy, tachycardia, and hypervolemia.
Respiratory system	Pulmonary edema, difficulty in breathing due to excess fluid, Kussmaul respiration due to metabolic acidosis.
Gastrointestinal system	Gastrointestinal bleeding, nausea and vomiting, loss of appetite due to uremia, metallic taste in the mouth, hiccup, and uremic halitosis.
Integumentary system	Uremic frost, pruritus, bruises, and pallor with edema.
Musculoskeletal system	Mineral bone disease or osteodystrophy.
Endocrine system	Hyperparathyroidism.
Immune system	High risk for immune suppression and infection.

Table 3.
Complication of CKD on multiple systems in body.

CKD is linked to various unfavorable clinical consequences, including cardiovascular events, mortality, and diminished quality of life [13]. **Table 3** explains the complication of CKD on system in the body function.

2. Pharmacological therapies for CKD in various stages

2.1 Mineralocorticoid receptor antagonist (MRA): Finerenone, spironolactone, eplerenone, esaxerenone, apararenone

Among the class of medications known as mineralocorticoid receptor antagonists (MRAs) are the classic steroid antagonists, spironolactone and eplerenone. We can differentiate between the nonsteroidal MRAs, such as apararenone, esaxerenone, and eplerenone [14]. Simpson et al. isolated aldosterone in 1953 [15]. The adrenal glands' glomerulosa cells are primarily responsible for producing it. The heart, blood arteries, and adipocytes can create aldosterone under specific conditions [16]. Human coronary arteries from multi-organ donors have demonstrated elevated expression of aldosterone synthetase (AS), which is also elevated in people suffering renal failure and coincides with the vascular expression of osteoblastic transforming factor: core-binding factor alpha 1 (CBFa1) [17].

In contrast to spironolactone or eplerenone, which is found primarily in the kidneys, the nonsteroidal MRA finerenone exhibits a balanced distribution between the heart and kidneys. Another important difference is that finerenone has a shorter half-life and no active metabolites, which may lessen its long-term impact on the sodium-potassium balance [18]. Despite a rise in hyperkalemia, classic mineralocorticoid receptor (MR) antagonists have been beneficial in reducing cardiovascular events and death in individuals with heart failure and reduced ejection fraction (EF). Activation of MR causes detrimental effects on the heart through several mechanisms that have been covered in this study. Nonsteroidal aldosterone antagonists may provide higher benefits in critical renal and cardiovascular variables due to their potential for increased cardiorenal protective capability and decreased risk of hyperkalemia. Two clinical trials involving finerenone will provide the definitive answer. The first trial, called FIDELIO-DKD (*Finerenone in reducing kidney failure and disease progression in diabetic kidney disease*), examines the effectiveness of finerenone in relation to placebo in reducing major renal and cardiovascular (CV) events in subjects with diabetes mellitus type 2 (DM-2) and chronic kidney disease (CKD) treated with angiotensin-converting enzyme inhibitor (ACEI) or angiotensin II receptor antagonists (ARA2) [19]. The second trial, called FIGARO-DKD (*Finerenone in reducing CV mortality and morbidity in diabetic kidney disease*), examines the safety and efficacy of finerenone in relation to placebo in patients with DM-2 and CKD [20].

2.2 Methylxanthine derivative: Pentoxifylline

Pentoxifylline (PTF) is a derivative of methylxanthine having a variety of pharmacologic actions, including immunological modulation, enhanced cellular membrane fluidity, fibrinolysis stimulation, anticoagulant effects, and altered fibroblast physiology [21]. PTF, a nonselective phosphodiesterase (PDE) inhibitor, has been shown to have strong inhibitory effects on the growth of cells, inflammation, and the buildup of extracellular matrix (ECM) [22]. It is widely accepted that PTF, by its hemorheological action as well as its anti-TNF α activity, can lessen proteinuria in diabetic individuals [23]. In a recent investigation on early-stage type 2 diabetic nephropathy, pentoxifylline was found to further decrease urine protein and N-acetyl-π-glucosaminidase excretion in patients receiving treatment with an ACE inhibitor or an angiotensin-receptor blocker (ARB) [24]. Based on these results, there is clinical evidence that PTF and renin-angiotensin-aldosterone system (RAAS) blockage together may further preserve kidney function.

Studies in humans and animals have shown that adding PTF to current CKD treatment might make it even better. In a randomized experiment conducted in 2012, the pharmacological therapy of 91 patients resulted in a one-year decrease in blood levels of fibrinogen, tumor necrosis factor α (TNF-α), and high-sensitivity C-reactive protein (hs-CRP), while eGFR rose by 2.4 mL/min/1.73 m^2 [25]. The results from this experiment demonstrated that 24 patients from the control group (13 started dialysis therapy and 11 had a twofold increase in serum creatinine) and 11 patients from the PTF group (seven started dialysis and four observed a double increase in serum creatinine) experienced renal events during follow-up. Irrespective of the existence of diabetes mellitus, the potential protective impact of PTF was more significant in individuals with albuminuria. PTF treatment decreased renal events by 35% as compared to the control group in a Cox model that incorporated basal renal function, albuminuria, and diabetes mellitus into account. With PTF therapy, cardiovascular mortality was considerably lower (2 patients vs. 10 in the control group). When age and diabetes mellitus were considered, PTF therapy decreased cardiovascular mortality by 55%. Another study has demonstrated that PTF administration lowers proteinuria and enhances renal function in people with chronic kidney disease [26]. In summary, PTF has been shown to have renoprotective properties in individuals with chronic kidney disease. To find out if PTF might improve renal outcomes in individuals undergoing proven-effective treatments, more clinical trials are required.

2.3 Glucagon-like peptide-1 (GLP-1) receptor agonists: Exenatide, lixisenatide, semaglutide, liraglutide

As a relatively recent class of antidiabetic medications, glucagon-like peptide-1 (GLP-1) receptor agonists are already in widespread usage. They modify the function of incretin GLP-1, a protein generated by small intestinal cells, by interfering with the GLP-1 receptor. By increasing glucose-dependent insulin secretion and decreasing glucagon secretion, stomach emptying, and food intake, this lowers HbA1c levels [27]. GLP-1 receptor agonists, in terms of CKD, play a role in lowering risk factors by reducing blood pressure, insulin, glucose, and inducing weight reduction [28]. The kidneys' GLP-1 receptor has been found in a few locations. Research carried out on animal models revealed that GLP-1 receptor messenger RiboNucleic Acid (mRNA) was expressed in the glomerulus and the first segment of the proximal convoluted tubes but not in any other area of the nephron [29]. GLP-1 receptors have also been detected in human kidneys, namely in proximal tubular cells and preglomerular vascular smooth muscle cells [30].

GLP-1 and GLP-1R agonists have been shown in experimental investigations to decrease renal RAAS activation indicators, such as angiotensin II levels and their detrimental effects on the glomerulus. These findings may point to additional possible renal protective mechanisms in diabetic kidney disease (DKD) [31]. Nevertheless, there is currently no solid data to support the impact of short- or long-term GLP-1R agonist therapy on circulating RAAS components. A little decrease in low-density lipoprotein levels is linked to inflammation in diabetes, according to GLP-1 receptor agonist treatment. Increased vascular inflammation and fibrosis have been linked to profibrotic growth factors, cytokines, and inflammatory cells in the pathophysiology of diabetic nephrotic (DN). GLP-1 affects inflammation at several places, including blood vessels and the kidneys, according to recent research [32]. It is possible to lower reactive oxygen species (ROS) generation in the diabetic kidney by activating the cyclic adenosine monophosphate–protein kinase A (cAMP–PKA) pathway. Since GLP-1 receptor activation stimulates the cAMP–PKA pathways, which have antioxidative properties, it is likely that GLP-1 shields the kidney from oxidative [33]. All of these results will serve as the foundation for the next clinical research examining whether GLP-1R agonists may enhance renal outcomes when DKD is present. SUSTAIN 6 (*Trial to Evaluate Cardiovascular and Other Long-term Outcomes With Semaglutide in Subjects With Type 2 Diabetes*) and LEADER (*Liraglutide Effect and Action in Diabetes*) were two randomized, double-blind, placebo-controlled studies that were carried out [34]. The benefits of once-weekly and once-daily semaglutide and liraglutide on several clinically significant kidney outcomes have been shown by analysis of these studies. These outcomes include changes in albuminuria, changes in the annual slope of the estimated glomerular filtration rate change, time to persistent proportional estimated glomerular filtration rate reductions of 40 and 50% from baseline, and a composite endpoint (time from randomization to first occurrence of kidney failure/death or proportional estimated glomerular filtration rate decline). The study's findings imply that patients with type 2 diabetes and diabetic kidney disease may have more alternatives for kidney-protective therapy if they take the glucagon-like peptide-1 receptor agonists such as semaglutide and liraglutide. Kidney Disease Improving Global Outcomes (KDIGO) recommends long-acting GLP-1 receptor agonists for patients with type 2 diabetes mellitus (T2DM) and chronic kidney disease (CKD) who have not reached individualized glycemic targets despite using metformin and SGLT2i treatment, or who are unable to use those medications [35].

2.4 Sodium-glucose cotransporter-2 (SGLT2) inhibitors: Empagliflozin, dapagliflozin, canagliflozin

Since the first SGLT2 inhibitor was introduced in 2012 [36], the class of drugs has expanded to include canagliflozin, dapagliflozin, empagliflozin, and ertugliflozin in the Americas and Europe, with other members of the class starting to gain traction in other areas [37]. SGLT2 inhibitors are glucose-lowering medications that decrease the renal filtrate's ability to absorb glucose, hence eliminating excess glucose through a glucosuric action [38]. Even though SGLT2 inhibitors have been developed to lower hyperglycemia and help with body weight control in people with type 2 diabetes, further therapeutic prospects for these drugs to treat the cardiorenal consequences and comorbidities of the disease are now identified. A growing number of research studies indicate that SGLT2 inhibitors can prevent DKD from developing and reduce the course of the condition both independently and in combination with RAAS inhibition.

The renal composite (doubling of serum creatinine, eGFR <45 ml/min/1.73 m^2, commencement of renal replacement therapy, or death from kidney disease) was 46% lower in the empagliflozin-treated groups in the EMPA-REG OUTCOME study [39]. According to the DECLARE-TIMI 58 study, dapagliflozin treatment was linked to a 47% lower renal composite of new end stage kidney disease (ESKD), mortality from renal cause, and a sustained drop in estimated glomerular filtration rate (eGFR) of ≥40% to <60 ml/min/1.73 m^2 [40]. Dapagliflozin was associated with a 46% reduction in eGFR decline (from >40% to <60 ml/min/1.73 m^2) as well as substantial reductions in ESKD and renal mortality. Dapagliflozin also reduced new-onset macroalbuminuria by 46% and new-onset albuminuria by 21% [41]. These study results demonstrate that SGLT2 inhibitors have a range of effects on the kidney, including acute and long-term nephroprotective effects that slow the progression of diabetic kidney disease and may even partially reverse its hallmark indicators. These effects are both directly and indirectly linked to decreased glucose reabsorption.

2.5 Pharmacological treatment using natural product for CKD in various stages

Plants, algae, and fungi have been used as natural remedies throughout history [42]. Natural products are regarded as an acceptable, cost-effective, readily available, and relatively safe source of many active pharmacological chemicals [43]. Many medicinal plants and their extracts have already been shown to improve kidney function *via* antioxidant action, with concomitant advantages for inflammation and fibrosis. For preclinical research, *in vitro* and *in vivo* tests with natural product-based medicines show some significant therapeutic advantages.

Wang et al. [44] found that Shen shuaining capsules containing *Rheum officinale*, *Radix pseudostellariae*, *Coptis chinensis*, *Carthamus tinctorius, the rhizome of Salvia miltiorrhiza*, and *Bidentate achyranthes* significantly reduced serum creatinine and blood urea nitrogen, increased hemoglobin, and improved overall efficacy of CKD symptoms and signs. A decoction of the roots of two Chinese herbs, *Astragalus membranaceus* and *Angelica sinensis*, has exhibited antifibrotic effects in rats with chronic kidney disorders and improved renal blood flow in rats with acute ischemic renal injury [45]. Aqueous extracts of *Fructus Corni* and *Radix Astragali* reduced urine protein levels and altered protein patterns, indicating that *Fructus Corni* and *Radix Astragali* could play a significant role in maintaining renal function in nephropathy mice [46].

Cordyceps sinensis and Tripterygium wilfordii polyglycosidium protected the podocytes of rats with diabetic nephropathy [47]. *Cordyceps cicadae* may inhibit renal fibrosis *in vivo* through the TGF-β1/CTGF pathway. According to the researchers, the usage of *Cordyceps cicadae* could provide a sensible strategy for fighting renal fibrosis [48]. *Elsholtzia ciliata* ethanol extract (ECE) may function by inhibiting the activation of TGF-ß and inflammatory cytokines, resulting in the breakdown of the extracellular matrix accumulation pathway. Based on these findings, ECE may be a more effective treatment for renal fibrosis [49].

Treatment with Azuki beans (an aqueous extract of *Vigna angularis*) improved renal function parameters and significantly reduced glucose levels, triglycerides, VLDL, alanine aminotransferase, uric acid, and creatinine, while also significantly increasing high-density lipoprotein (HDL) levels in rats subjected to a model of moderate chronic kidney disease [50]. Shenkang granules (SKGs) are a Chinese herbal medicinal formula consisting of rhubarb (*Rheum palmatum*), *Salvia miltiorrhiza*, milkvetch root (*Astragalus membranaceus*), and safflower (*Carthamus tinctorius* L.). SKG was shown to reduce renal damage in a rat model of chronic renal failure (CRF). Thus, SKG may have a positive therapeutic effect on CRF [51].

The hydro-ethanolic extract of *Euphorbia neriifolia* significantly restored antioxidant enzyme levels in the kidney and demonstrated a significant dose-dependent protective effect against N-nitrosodiethylamine-induced nephrotoxicity, which can be attributed primarily to the extract's antioxidant properties [52]. The hydroalcoholic extract of Rubia cordifolia roots (HARC) protects against ethylene glycol-induced urolithiasis by reducing and inhibiting the formation of urinary stones. As a result, HARC can help prevent the condition from recurring because it has been shown to influence the early stages of stone growth. The mechanism underlying this benefit may be mediated by an antioxidant, nephroprotection, and its influence on urinary stone-forming ingredients and risk factors [53]. *Aunaea procumbens* efficiently protects rats' kidneys from CCl_4-induced oxidative damage *via* the antioxidant and free radical scavenging properties of flavonoids and saponins in the fractions [54]. Another study reported that grape seed extract reduced inflammation by lowering CRP and triglyceridemia while counteracting anemia and thrombocytopenia. Supplementation with 2 g GSE/day for 6 months improved various kidney function parameters in CKD patients, and this therapeutic effect of Grape seed extract appears to be mediated at least partially by its antioxidant and anti-inflammatory characteristics [55]. Jimenez-Osorio et al. [42] reported that curcumin administration lowers oxidative stress in Mexican patients with nondiabetic or diabetic proteinuric CKD.

There is no disagreement that natural products represent a significant untapped source of novel CKD therapy. Clinical and preclinical trials of plant extracts have occasionally shown benefits; however, some research has also shown that plant extracts can cause chronic organ dysfunction when administered over time due to the presence of toxic compounds. Natural products are frequently regarded as safer than standard drugs, and many of our current medications are developed from herbs. Nonetheless, several researchers are concerned about their safe use.

2.6 Management of CKD patients in stage 4 and stage 5

2.6.1 Renal replacement therapy

Renal replacement therapy (RRT) is a medical intervention that substitutes the essential functions of the kidneys in individuals with severe kidney failure of End-stage renal disease (ESRD). This therapy is necessary when the kidneys are no longer able to adequately filter waste products and excess fluids from the blood [56]. The three modalities of RRT are hemodialysis, peritoneal dialysis, and kidney transplantation. The choice of treatment is the patient's preference and according to their condition.

2.7 Hemodialysis

Hemodialysis is a complex procedure for renal failure patients that require frequent dialysis center visits or hospitalizations that may be encountered 3 to 4 times per week [57]. The goal of dialysis is to remove the end product of protein metabolism from the blood. Maintain a safe concentration of serum electrolytes. Correct the acidosis, replenish the body's bicarbonate buffer system, and remove excess fluid from the blood. Hemodialysis is needed when the eGFR drops below 20 ml/min/1.73 m^2 or when there is a rapid progression of kidney disease to end-stage renal disease. Gotch and Sargent established the Kt/V urea as a measure in their National Cooperative Dialysis study (1985). In contrast to a Kt/V of more than 1.0, which resulted in a favorable outcome, it was shown that Kt/V of less than 0.8 was linked to increased morbidity or treatment failure [58].

It is a dimensionless ratio calculated by dividing the amount of plasma cleared of urea (Kt) by the distribution volume of urea (V). The urea-free plasma volume is the product of blood urea clearance (K) and dialysis session length (t). A Kt/V ratio of 1.0 indicates that the total blood volume cleansed during a session equals the urea distribution volume. Dialysis can be intermittent or continuous. Continuous intravascular procedures are preferred for patients who are hemodynamically unstable or have a high-volume overload. A dialyzer will connect the circuits. Side ports in the veins are used for saline or heparin infusion, air entrance detection, and pressure measurement. The dialysate is pushed through the dialysate compartment which is isolated from the blood compartment by the dialyzer's semi-permeable membrane. Regenerated cellulose, with its very hydrophilic character, permits miniaturization of the dialyzer and lower membrane thickness. Biocompatible synthetic membranes composed of polysulfone have a semi-permeable surface and lower complement cascade activation than previous bioincompatible ones. The temperature and concentration of dissolved components in dialysis fluid are controlled. A blood leak detector pauses dialysis when it detects blood products in the outflow dialysate. Approximately 25% of patients having uremia need hospital administration for the procedure preparation and management of complications. The distal arteriovenous (AV) fistula serves as the gold standard for hemodialysis access. If the patients' superficial veins are exhausted, the alternative methods will be intrajugular cannulation (IJC), femoral catheter, permanent catheter, and synthetic graft. Patients that need to undergo dialysis treatment can make appointments in the dialysis unit and schedule their time according to their daily routine. Some of the patients will need three times per week [59].

2.8 Peritoneal dialysis

This is another type of renal replacement therapy that uses the patient's own peritoneum cavity as a natural permeable membrane that allows water and solutes to equilibrate [60]. Peritoneal dialysis is a more suggested procedure for patients than hemodialysis due to less physiological stress, does not require vascular access, and can be done at home, and the patients have more flexibility. Although this is the most suggested procedure, it still needs more patient involvement than in-center hemodialysis. The sterile technique is very important for this procedure. Two processes involved in this procedure are osmosis and diffusion. In this procedure, the usage of dialysate is the mainstay for the dialysis, and it is instilled using a Tenckhoff catheter. Peritoneal dialysis can be done manually or by using an automated device [61].

Manual methods of peritoneal dialysis include:

- Continuous ambulatory peritoneal dialysis (CAPD) that does not require a machine for exchange. For an adult, approximately 2 to 3 L of dialysate can be used four to five times per day. Dialysate is a glucose solution for the process of osmosis.

- Intermittent peritoneal dialysis is used for immediate management of acute kidney injury. Warm dialysate will be instilled for 10 to 15 minutes. Frequent exchange will be needed for almost 12 to 48 hours.

Using machines for peritoneal dialysis are as follows:

- Continuous cyclic peritoneal dialysis (CCPD) will need 12 to 5 hours of dwelling time and 3 to 6 nighttime exchanges using automated cycler.

- Noctural intermittent peritoneal dialysis (NIPD) will need nighttime exchange, and the patient will not need daytime exchange.

- Tidal peritoneal dialysis involves the remaining dialysate fluid in the peritoneum for one exchange to another, which may allay frequent repositioning.

Although peritoneal dialysis is a recommended procedure, it still can be a failure for patients if an aseptic technique is not applied. Therefore, all the patients with peritoneal dialysis will be given training and health education to maintain the aseptic technique and adhere to the procedure without the main complication, which is peritonitis [62].

3. Renal transplant

It is known that when a CKD patient has been scheduled for a kidney transplant, they are considered to have a gift of life. Patients that have 10–15% of remaining kidney function are known to be in the condition of end-stage renal disease (ESRD), and kidney transplant is performed to prolong and improve the quality of life (QOL) for them [63]. This surgery has been developed for over 50 years. This procedure has better long-term survival. There is evidence that patients undergoing renal transplants have survived more than 10 years. The first renal transplant was successfully conducted by Dr. Joseph Murray in 1954with major development in immunology and transplant procedure. If the patients have no contraindications, the nephrologist will refer the patients for transplant workup plan. There is a clear survival benefit for kidney transplant recipients over those who remain on dialysis.

There are many complications and comorbidities from kidney disease for ESRD patients. Therefore, careful screening is needed for both donor and recipient. They will need to undergo investigation such as cardiovascular assessment, renal angiogram, human leukocyte antigen (HLA) compatibility, cerebellar vascular disease screening, frailty test, gastrointestinal evaluation, hematologic disease screening, infectious disease screening, and pulmonary assessment. There are three types of kidney donors: living-related donor, living nonrelated donor, and cadaveric donor [64]. Living related can be parents, siblings, and other blood-related. Living nonrelated can be husband and wife or friends, and cadaveric donor is the deceased donor that is broken down to brain death.

Currently, there is robotic surgery for transplants. Access is achieved to the intraperitoneal space to insert the port. The left kidney's ureter and gonadal vein are discovered at the pelvic brim after the left colon is released from peritoneal attachments and tracked cephalad to locate and isolate the renal vein and artery [65]. The adrenal gland is separated from the upper pole of the kidney, and the adrenal vein has been divided. Once the kidney is fully mobilized and only connected by the artery, vein, and ureter, a slightly bigger incision is created to prepare for rapid extraction. The distal ureter is divided with clips, and the hilar arteries are separated with a laparoscopic vascular-load stapler. Some changes in dissection exist depending on which kidney is obtained. To access the right kidney, the liver is retracted, and the right colon and duodenum are partially mobilized. Following extraction, the organ is moved off the pitch and ready for implantation on the back table.

The open surgical approach for living donor procurement involves making a subcostal incision and exposing the retroperitoneal region. Before extraction, the ureter is followed down to the iliac vessels, where it is split. The kidney will be isolated on its vascular pedicle, and when the recipient team is ready, the renal artery and vein are transacted before the organ is transferred. The tributary stumps are then ligatured or oversewn. The remaining perinephric fat is trimmed while the kidney is prepared for implantation.

Patients with CKD and ESRD depend on hemodialysis and peritoneal dialysis before the initiation of the transplant. Once the transplant was set in gear, the survival rate of ESRD patients increased. Those who went for renal transplants experienced a better quality of life than those on dialysis treatment. CKD, concomitant diseases, and its treatment impose significant burdens on patients' health-related quality of life. Kidney illness, including polycystic kidney disease and nephrotic syndrome, is associated with significant QOL impairment.

4. Quality of life for CKD patients'

Monitoring patient-reported outcomes to capture CKD's effect on health-related quality of life (QOL) is critical for both population and individual care. Patients with CKD require more practice and clinically relevant patient-reported outcome measures [66]. QOL declines with increasing CKD severity; patients at earlier CKD stages have smaller but still significant QOL impairments compared to the general and hypertensive populations. Those patients with CKD stage 5 who are about to start dialysis report physical health lower than the general population.

4.1 Methods to increase CKD patients' quality of life

1. *Education and empowerment* provides comprehensive education about CKD including its cause, progression, treatment options, and self-management strategies. Empowering patients with knowledge helps them make informed decisions and actively participate in their care.

2. *Dietary management* can collaborate with a registered dietitian to develop a personalized nutrition plan that addresses the patient's specific dietary needs including restrictions on sodium, potassium, phosphorus, and protein intake. A well-balanced diet tailored to CKD can help manage symptoms and slow disease progression.

3. *Physical activity* is needed, and it should be within the patients' capabilities. Exercise can improve cardiovascular health, muscle strength, and overall well-being. Recommend activities such as walking, swimming, or light resistance training, considering the individual's fitness and any physical limitations.

4. *Medication adherence* by ensuring that patients adhere to their prescribed medication regimen, including medications to control blood pressure, manage symptoms, and treat comorbid conditions such as diabetes or cardiovascular disease. Monitor for any adverse effects and adjust medications as needed.

5. *Symptom management* by identifying fatigue, nausea, itching, and pain through appropriate interventions, including medication adjustments, lifestyle modifications, and supportive therapies. Managing symptoms effectively can enhance the patient's comfort and quality of life.

6. *Psychological support* is important to recognize and address the emotional impact of CKD, which may include anxiety, depression, stress, and adjustment difficulties. Offer psychological support through counseling, support groups, or referrals to mental health professionals.

7. *Social support and community engagement* by fostering connections and encouraging participants in support groups or community activities. Social support can provide emotional comfort, practical assistance, and opportunities for socialization, which are essential for maintaining overall well-being.

8. *Palliative care and hospice service* can be considered for patients with advanced CKD, focusing on symptom management, pain relief, and improving the quality of life. These services provide comprehensive support for patients and their families during the end-of-life stage.

9. *Advanced care planning* facilitates discussions about advanced care planning to help patients articulate their healthcare preferences, values, and goals of care. Advance directives, including living wills and surfable power of attorney for healthcare, ensure that patient's wishes are honored, particularly in critical or end-of-life situations.

10. *Regular monitoring and follow-up* are needed to monitor kidney function, assess treatment efficacy, and address any concerns or complications promptly. Close monitoring allows for timely adjustments to the treatment plan, optimizing outcomes and quality of life.

11. *Financial assistance and resources* will provide information about financial assistance programs, insurance coverage options, and community resources available to support CKD patients in managing the financial aspects of their care. Access to affordable healthcare and medication is crucial for improving quality of life and treatment adherence.

By implementing these strategies, healthcare providers can effectively enhance the quality of life for CKD patients and support them in managing their condition.

5. Conclusion

This book chapter delves into the intricate landscape of chronic kidney disease (CKD), offering a comprehensive exploration of its multifaceted dimensions. Through a meticulous examination of the underlying causes, diagnostic criteria, and progression of CKD, we have gained valuable insights into the complex interplay of genetic, environmental, and lifestyle factors that contribute to its development. Furthermore, the discussion on the various stages of CKD underscores the importance of detection and intervention, emphasizing the potential for preventive measures to mitigate the advancement of this silent yet pervasive condition. The nuanced exploration of treatment modalities, including pharmacological interventions and lifestyle modifications, highlights the evolving landscape of CKD management and the promising avenues for improving patients' outcomes. As we navigate the intricate web of complications associated with CKD, ranging from cardiovascular issues to metabolic alterations, a holistic approach to patient care emerges as a central theme. The integration of multidisciplinary strategies, encompassing nephrology, cardiology, endocrinology, and lifestyle interventions, underscores the imperative of a collaborative and patient-centered paradigm.

Moreover, this chapter not only serves as a valuable resource for healthcare professionals but also empowers patients with the knowledge to actively engage in their journey toward optimal kidney health. This exploration of CKD contributes to the ongoing discourse on public health initiatives, emphasizing the need for early detection, preventive measures, and comprehensive management strategies to alleviate the burden of CKD on individuals and healthcare system alike. As we continue to unravel the complexities of CKD, this chapter serves as a stepping stone to a deeper understanding and more effective management of the pervasive health challenge.

Author details

Kogila Supramanian[1*], Mahendran Sekar[2] and Nor Safwan Hadi Nor Afendi[3]

1 Faculty of Medicine, Nursing Department, Universiti Kuala Lumpur, Royal College of Medicine Perak, Ipoh, Perak, Malaysia

2 School of Pharmacy, Monash University Malaysia, Bandar Sunway, Selangor, Malaysia

3 Faculty of Pharmacy and Health Science, Universiti Kuala Lumpur, Royal College of Medicine Perak, Ipoh, Perak, Malaysia

*Address all correspondence to: kogila@unikl.edu.my

References

[1] Inker LA, Astor BC, Fox CH, Isakova T, Lash JP, Peralta CA, et al. KDOQI US commentary on the 2012 KDIGO clinical practice guideline for the evaluation and management of CKD. American Journal of Kidney Diseases. 2014;**63**(5):713-735

[2] Webster AC, Nagler EV, Morton RL, Masson P. Chronic Kidney Disease. Lancet. 25 Mar 2017;**389**(10075):1238-1252

[3] Daugirdas JT, Depner TA, Inrig J, Mehrotra R, Rocco MV, Suri RS, et al. KDOQI clinical practice guideline for hemodialysis adequacy: 2015 update. American Journal of Kidney Diseases. 2015;**66**(5):884-930

[4] Yu HT. Progression of chronic renal failure. Archives of Internal Medicine. 2003;**163**(12):1417-1429. DOI: 10.1001/archinte.163.12.1417

[5] Methven S, Traynor JP, Hair MD, O'Reilly St. J, Deighan CJ, MacGregor MS. Stratifying risk in chronic kidney disease: An observational study of UK guidelines for measuring total proteinuria and albuminuria. QJM. 2011;**104**(8):663-670. DOI: 10.1093/qjmed/hcr026. Epub 2011 Mar 7

[6] Hallan SI, Orth SR. Smoking is a risk factor in the progression to kidney failure. Kidney International. 2011;**80**(5):516-523. DOI: 10.1038/ki.2011.157

[7] de Brito-Ashurst I, Varagunam M, Raftery MJ, Yaqoob MM. Bicarbonate supplementation slows progression of CKD and improves nutritional status. Journal of the American Society of Nephrology. 2009;**20**(9):2075-2084. DOI: 10.1681/ASN.2008111205

[8] Alshahrani S. Renin–angiotensin–aldosterone pathway modulators in chronic kidney disease: A comparative review. Frontiers in Pharmacology. 2023;**14**:1101068

[9] Schnaper HW. Remnant nephron physiology and the progression of chronic kidney disease. Pediatric Nephrology. 2014;**29**:193-202

[10] Levin A, Stevens PE, Bilous RW, Coresh J, De Francisco AL, De Jong PE, et al. Kidney disease: Improving global outcomes (KDIGO) CKD work group. KDIGO 2012 clinical practice guideline for the evaluation and management of chronic kidney disease. Kidney International Supplements. 2013;**3**(1):1-50

[11] Wheeler DC, Becker GJ. Summary of KDIGO guideline. What do we really know about management of blood pressure in patients with chronic kidney disease? Kidney International. 2013;**83**(3):377-383

[12] de Boer IH, Caramori ML, Chan JC, Heerspink HJ, Hurst C, Khunti K, et al. KDIGO 2020 clinical practice guideline for diabetes management in chronic kidney disease. Kidney International. 2020;**98**(4):S1-S15

[13] Bello AK, Alrukhaimi M, Ashuntantang GE, Basnet S, Rotter RC, Douthat WG, et al. Complications of chronic kidney disease: Current state, knowledge gaps, and strategy for action. Kidney International Supplements. 2017;**7**(2):122-129

[14] Erraez S, López-Mesa M, Gómez-Fernández P. Bloqueantes del receptor mineralcorticoide en la enfermedad renal crónica. Nefrología.

2021;**41**(3):258-275. DOI: 10.1016/j.nefro.2020.10.001

[15] Cat AND, Friederich-Persson M, White A, Touyz RM. Adipocytes, aldosterone and obesity-related hypertension. Journal of Molecular Endocrinology. 2016;**57**(1):F7-F21. DOI: 10.1530/JME-16-0025

[16] Barrera-Chimal J, Jaisser F, Anders H-J. The mineralocorticoid receptor in chronic kidney disease. British Journal of Pharmacology. 2022;**179**(13):3152-3164. DOI: 10.1111/bph.15734

[17] Ruilope LM, Agarwal R, Anker SD, Bakris GL, Filippatos G, Nowack C, et al. Design and baseline characteristics of the finerenone in reducing cardiovascular mortality and morbidity in diabetic kidney disease trial. American Journal of Nephrology. 2019;**50**(5):345-356. DOI: 10.1159/000503712

[18] Simpson SA, Tait JF, Wettstein A, Neher R, Von Euw J, Reichstein T. Isolation from the adrenals of a new crystalline hormone with especially high effectiveness on mineral metabolism. Experientia. 1953;**9**(9):333-335. DOI: 10.1007/BF02155834

[19] Alesutan I, Voelkl J, Feger M, Kratschmar DV, Castor T, Mia S, et al. Involvement of vascular aldosterone synthase in phosphate-induced osteogenic transformation of vascular smooth muscle cells. Scientific Reports. 2017;**7**(1):1-15. DOI: 10.1038/s41598-017-01882-2

[20] Bakris GL, Agarwal R, Anker SD, Pitt B, Ruilope LM, Nowack C, et al. Design and baseline characteristics of the Finerenone in reducing kidney failure and disease progression in diabetic kidney disease trial. American Journal of Nephrology. 2019;**50**(5):333-344. DOI: 10.1159/000503713

[21] Samlaska CP, Winfield EA. Pentoxifylline. Journal of the American Academy of Dermatology. 1994;**30**(4):603-621. DOI: 10.1016/S0190-9622(94)70069-9

[22] Lin SL, Chiang WC, Chen YM, Lai CF, Tsai TJ, Hsieh BS. The renoprotective potential of pentoxifylline in chronic kidney disease. Journal of the Chinese Medical Association. 2005;**68**(3):99-105. DOI: 10.1016/S1726-4901(09)70228-X

[23] Solerte SB, Fioravanti M, Bozzetti A, Schifino N, Patti AL, Fedele P, et al. Pentoxifylline, albumin excretion rate and proteinuria in type I and type II diabetic patients with microproteinuria. Results of a short-term randomized study. Acta Diabetologica Latina. 1986;**23**(2):171-177. DOI: 10.1007/BF02624677

[24] Navarro JF, Mora C, Muros M, Maca M, Garca J. Effects of pentoxifylline administration on urinary N-acetyl-beta-glucosaminidase excretion in type 2 diabetic patients: A short-term, prospective, randomized study. American Journal of Kidney Diseases : The Official Journal of the National Kidney Foundation. 2003;**42**(2):264-270. DOI: 10.1016/s0272-6386(03)00651-6

[25] de Morales AM, Goicoechea M, Verde E, Carbayo J, Barbieri D, Delgado A, et al. Pentoxifylline, progression of chronic kidney disease (CKD) and cardiovascular mortality: Long-term follow-up of a randomized clinical trial. Journal of Nephrology. 2019;**32**(4):581-587. DOI: 10.1007/s40620-019-00607-0

[26] Jiang X, Zhou S, Yao J, Kong X, Cui M. Effect of pentoxifylline in proteinuric chronic kidney disease: A systematic review and meta-analysis.

Journal of Nephrology. 2016;**29**(5):653-662. DOI: 10.1007/s40620-015-0240-y

[27] Zhao X, Wang M, Wen Z, Lu Z, Cui L, Fu C, et al. GLP-1 Receptor Agonists: Beyond Their Pancreatic Effects. Frontiers in Endocrinology. 23 Aug 2021;**12**:721135. DOI: 10.3389/fendo.2021.721135

[28] Greco EV, Russo G, Giandalia A, Viazzi F, Pontremoli R, De Cosmo S. GLP-1 receptor agonists and kidney protection. Medicina (Lithuania). 2019;**55**(6):1-14. DOI: 10.3390/medicina55060233

[29] Crajoinas RO, Oricchio FT, Pessoa TD, Pacheco BPM, Lessa LMA, Malnic G, et al. Mechanisms mediating the diuretic and natriuretic actions of the incretin hormone glucagon-like peptide-1. American Journal of Physiology - Renal Physiology. 2011;**301**(2):355-363. DOI: 10.1152/ajprenal.00729.2010

[30] Pyke C, Heller RS, Kirk RK, Ørskov C, Reedtz-Runge S, Kaastrup P, et al. GLP-1 receptor localization in monkey and human tissue: Novel distribution revealed with extensively validated monoclonal antibody. Endocrinology. 2014;**155**(4):1280-1290. DOI: 10.1210/en.2013-1934

[31] Roscioni SS, Heerspink HJL, De Zeeuw D. The effect of RAAS blockade on the progression of diabetic nephropathy. Nature Reviews Nephrology. 2014;**10**(2):77-87. DOI: 10.1038/nrneph.2013.251

[32] Lee YS, Jun HS. Anti-inflammatory effects of GLP-1-based therapies beyond glucose control. Mediators of Inflammation. 2016;**2016**:26-32. DOI: 10.1155/2016/3094642

[33] Deb DK, Bao R, Li YC. Critical role of the cAMP-PKA pathway in hyperglycemia-induced epigenetic activation of fibrogenic program in the kidney. The FASEB Journal. 2017;**31**(5):2065-2075. DOI: 10.1096/fj.201601116R

[34] Shaman AM, Bain SC, Bakris GL, Buse JB, Idorn T, Mahaffey KW, et al. Effect of the glucagon-like Peptide-1 receptor agonists Semaglutide and Liraglutide on kidney outcomes in patients with type 2 diabetes: Pooled analysis of SUSTAIN 6 and LEADER. Circulation. 2022;**145**(8):575-585. DOI: 10.1161/CIRCULATIONAHA.121.055459

[35] International, K. KDIGO 2022 clinical practice guideline for diabetes Management in chronic kidney disease. Kidney International. 2022;**102**(5):S1-S127. DOI: 10.1016/j.kint.2022.06.008

[36] Imamura M, Nakanishi K, Suzuki T, Ikegai K, Shiraki R, Ogiyama T, et al. Discovery of Ipragliflozin (ASP1941): A novel C-glucoside with benzothiophene structure as a potent and selective sodium glucose co-transporter 2 (SGLT2) inhibitor for the treatment of type 2 diabetes mellitus. Bioorganic & Medicinal Chemistry. 2012;**20**(10):3263-3279. DOI: 10.1016/j.bmc.2012.03.051

[37] Bailey CJ, Day C, Bellary S. Renal protection with SGLT2 inhibitors: Effects in acute and chronic kidney disease. Current Diabetes Reports. 2022;**22**(1):39-52. DOI: 10.1007/s11892-021-01442-z

[38] Ghezzi C, Loo DDF, Wright EM. Physiology of renal glucose handling via SGLT1, SGLT2 and GLUT2. Diabetologia. 2018;**61**(10):2087-2097. DOI: 10.1007/s00125-018-4656-5

[39] Wanner C, Inzucchi SE, Lachin JM, Fitchett D, von Eynatten M, Mattheus M, et al. Empagliflozin and progression of kidney disease in type 2 diabetes.

New England Journal of Medicine. 2016;**375**(4):323-334. DOI: 10.1056/nejmoa1515920

[40] Wiviott SD, Raz I, Bonaca MP, Mosenzon O, Kato ET, Cahn A, et al. Dapagliflozin and cardiovascular outcomes in type 2 diabetes. New England Journal of Medicine. 2019;**380**(4):347-357. DOI: 10.1056/nejmoa181238

[41] Mosenzon O, Wiviott SD, Cahn A, Rozenberg A, Yanuv I, Goodrich EL, et al. Effects of dapagliflozin on development and progression of kidney disease in patients with type 2 diabetes: An analysis from the DECLARE–TIMI 58 randomised trial. The Lancet Diabetes and Endocrinology. 2019;7(8):606-617. DOI: 10.1016/S2213-8587(19)30180-9

[42] Jiménez-Osorio AS, García-Niño WR, González-Reyes S, Álvarez-Mejía AE, Guerra-León S, Salazar-Segovia J, et al. The effect of dietary supplementation with curcumin on redox status and Nrf2 activation in patients with nondiabetic or diabetic Proteinuric chronic kidney disease: A pilot study. Journal of Renal Nutrition. 2016;**26**(4):237-244

[43] Turki K, Charradi K, Boukhalfa H, Belhaj M, Limam F, Aouani E. Grape seed powder improves renal failure of chronic kidney disease patients. EXCLI Journal. 2016;**15**:424-433

[44] Khan RA, Khan MR, Sahreen S. Evaluation of Launaea procumbens use in renal disorders: A rat model. Journal of Ethnopharmacology. 2010;**128**(2):452-461

[45] Divakar K, Pawar AT, Chandrasekhar SB, Dighe SB, Divakar G. Protective effect of the hydro-alcoholic extract of Rubia cordifolia roots against ethylene glycol induced urolithiasis in rats. Food and Chemical Toxicology. 2010;**48**(4):1013-1018

[46] Pracheta P, Sharma V, Singh L, Paliwal R, Sharma S, Yadav S, et al. Chemopreventive effect of hydroethanolic extract of Euphorbia neriifolia leaves against DENA-induced renal carcinogenesis in mice. Asian Pacific Journal of Cancer Prevention. 2011;**12**(3):677-683

[47] Zhang YU, Zhou N, Wang H, Wang S, He J. Effect of Shenkang granules on the progression of chronic renal failure in 5/6 nephrectomized rats. Experimental and Therapeutic Medicine. 2015;**9**(6):2034-2042

[48] Baracho NC, Monteiro NF, Borges MG, Arguelho RR. Effect of aqueous extract of the Vigna angularis in rats subjected to an experimental model of moderate chronic kidney disease. Acta Cirúrgica Brasileira. 2016;**31**(8):527-532

[49] Kim TW, Kim YJ, Seo CS, Kim HT, Park SR, Lee MY, et al. Elsholtzia ciliata (Thunb.) Hylander attenuates renal inflammation and interstitial fibrosis via regulation of TGF-ß and Smad3 expression on unilateral ureteral obstruction rat model. Phytomedicine. 2016;**23**(4):331-339

[50] Zhu R, Chen YP, Deng YY, Zheng R, Zhong YF, Wang L, et al. Cordyceps cicadae extracts ameliorate renal malfunction in a remnant kidney model. Journal of Zhejiang University. Science. B. 2011;**12**(12):1024-1033

[51] Hao L, Pan MS, Zheng Y, Wang RF. Effect of *Cordyceps sinensis* and *Tripterygium wilfordii* polyglycosidium on podocytes in rats with diabetic nephropathy. Experimental and Therapeutic Medicine. 2014;**7**(6):1465-1470

[52] Meng L, Qu L, Tang J, Cai SQ, Wang H, Li X. A combination of Chinese herbs, Astragalus membranaceus var.

mongholicus and Angelica sinensis, enhanced nitric oxide production in obstructed rat kidney. Vascular Pharmacology. 2007;**47**(2-3):174-183

[53] Wang S, Zhang J, Guo M, Lian X, Sun M, Guo L. The efficacy of Shen Shuaining capsule on chronic kidney disease: A systematic review and meta-analysis. Evidence-based Complementary and Alternative Medicine. 2016;**2016**:7515413

[54] Zhong Y et al. Recent advances in traditional Chinese medicine for kidney disease. American Journal of Kidney Diseases. 2015;**66**(3):513-522

[55] Gobe GC, Wojcikowski K. Nontraditional (non-Western pharmaceutical) treatments for chronic kidney disease. Clinical Nephrology. 2019;**93**(1):49-54

[56] Villa G, Ricci Z, Ronco C. Renal replacement therapy. Critical Care Clinics. 2015;**31**(4):839-848

[57] Mallick NP, Gokal RJ. Haemodialysis. The Lancet. 1999;**353**(9154):737-742

[58] Ronco C, Clark WR. Haemodialysis membranes. Nature Reviews Nephrology. 2018;**14**(6):394-410

[59] Bello AK, Okpechi IG, Osman MA, Cho Y, Htay H, Jha V, et al. Epidemiology of haemodialysis outcomes. Nature Reviews Nephrology. 2022;**18**(6):378-395

[60] Gokal R, Mallick NP. Peritoneal dialysis. The Lancet. 1999;**353**(9155): 823-828

[61] Teitelbaum I, Burkart J. Peritoneal dialysis. American Journal of Kidney Diseases. 2003;**42**(5):1082-1096

[62] Andreoli MC, Totoli C. Peritoneal dialysis. Revista da Associação Médica Brasileira. 2020;**66**:s37-s44

[63] Suthanthiran M, Strom TB. Renal transplantation. New England Journal of Medicine. 1994;**331**(6):365-376

[64] Thiruchelvam PT, Willicombe M, Hakim N, Taube D, Papalois V. Renal transplantation. BMJ. 2011;**343**

[65] Perrone RD, Coons SJ, Cavanaugh K, Finkelstein F, Meyer KB. Patient-reported outcomes in clinical trials of CKD-related therapies: Report of a symposium sponsored by the National Kidney Foundation and the US Food and Drug Administration. American Journal of Kidney Diseases. 2013;**62**(6):1046-1057

[66] Da Silva-Gane M, Wellsted D, Greenshields H, Norton S, Chandna SM, Farrington K. Quality of life and survival in patients with advanced kidney failure managed conservatively or by dialysis. Clinical Journal of the American Society of Nephrology. 2012;7:2002-2009

Chapter 3

Epithelial TGF-β/β-Catenin Axis in Proximal Tubule Response to Chronic Kidney Disease

Stellor Nlandu Khodo

Abstract

Chronic kidney disease (CKD) affects 10% of humans and increases the risk of cardiovascular diseases. Regardless of the etiology, tubulointerstitial fibrosis (TIF) is the histopathological feature of CKD that correlates with the loss of renal function, and excessive growth factor (GF) activation is a common mechanism in CKD. Among several GF pathways, the TGF-β/β-catenin axis plays a crucial role in the pathophysiology of CKD. Most compelling studies reported the pivotal role of the proximal tubule (PT), the most metabolic and vulnerable renal segment, in the post-injury response and the pathogenesis of CKD. Though the systemic activation of the TGF-β/β-catenin axis is detrimental in CKD, recent studies have reported the beneficial effects of the TGF-β/β-catenin axis in the PT's response to chronic injury. This chapter describes the recent findings on the role of TGF-β/β-catenin axis in the PT's response to CKD. Using genetically modified mice and biochemical and microscopy techniques, TGF-β/β-catenin axis revealed promoting mitochondrial homeostasis, regenerative Th1 immune response, G1 cell arrest, and survival. Future experimental studies should identify key downstream effectors in this axis that can be targeted to mitigate CKD progression.

Keywords: chronic kidney disease, epithelial TGF-β signaling, epithelial β-catenin signaling, proximal mitochondria and metabolism, Th1 immune response, cell cycle arrest

1. Introduction

Fibrosis or accumulation of extracellular matrix (ECM) proteins is a common pathological feature of progressive chronic diseases. Regardless of the organ, most therapeutic strategies fail to impede the progression of fibrosis and organ loss of function [1–3]. Tubulointerstitial fibrosis (TIF), the hallmark of chronic kidney disease (CKD), affects more than 10% of humans worldwide and increases the risk of cardiovascular diseases and stroke [4–8]. CKD treatment represents a considerable financial burden that threatens global health care systems [9–11]. Though our understanding of mechanisms involved in TIF progression has improved in the last few decades, a curative treatment for CKD patients is still out of reach in practice. Excessive transforming growth factor-beta (TGF-β) and Wnt/β-catenin activation signaling are two common features in CKD progression [12, 13]. Several studies demonstrated the beneficial effect of systemic inhibition of TGF-β signaling in mouse models of TIF; however, genetic inhibition of TGF-β signaling in the renal epithelia and matrix-producing interstitial cells (MPICs) did not mitigate TIF progression [14, 15]. Moreover, Voelker J et al. demonstrated that the addition of TGF-β1 monoclonal antibody to renin-angiotensin system (RAS) inhibitors did not slow the progression of diabetic nephropathy, suggesting that TGF-β signaling is not exclusively the main driving force in CKD progression [3]. Recently, experimental studies in mice demonstrated that deletion of the TGF-β type II receptor (*TbRII*) in the proximal tubule (PT), the most metabolic renal segment, aggravates TIF in two models of CKD mimicking toxin-induced (aristolochic acid nephrotoxicity) and hypertensive (uninephrectomy/angiotensin 2) nephropathies, implying a possible beneficial effect of epithelial TGF-β signaling in chronic tubular injury [16–19]. Wnt/β-catenin pathway is upregulated in biopsies of human diabetic kidneys and in the PT of proteinuric human patients. Several studies have shown the profibrotic effect of Wnt/β-catenin in fibroblasts/pericytes, but not in renal epithelia [20–24]. Recently, compelling data demonstrated the beneficial effect of constitutive active β-catenin stabilization in the PT upon chronic tubular injury [18, 25].

The PT is the most sensitive renal segment to injury partly due to its high metabolic rate, oxygen dependency, and higher exposure to toxins. Upon injury, PT cells sense their substratum integrity, undergo cell-autonomous mechanisms, and secrete growth factors/cytokines that activate renal interstitial cells to complete the post-injury recovery [26]. Unfortunately, this tubulointerstitial crosstalk usually becomes maladaptive under chronic injury, leading to TIF. Though the reparative capacity of the PT is incontestable, the mechanisms and molecular signature underlying this process are still elusive. This chapter recapitulates the most recent knowledge on how the TGF-β/β-catenin axis mediates PT adaptive response to chronic injury.

2. Renal tubulointerstitial fibrosis (TIF)

Fibrosis is a pathological condition characterized by the accumulation of extracellular matrix (ECM) proteins including collagens, fibronectin, and vimentin. TIF is the common pathological feature of late-stage renal diseases associated with progressive loss of renal function. The histopathological features of TIF are notable ECM protein accumulation in association with immune cell infiltration, tubular cell loss, myofibroblast proliferation, and rarefaction of micro-vessels. Multiple mechanisms including chronic inflammation, hypoxia, oxidative stress, cell reprogramming, and excessive growth factor activity intertwine in the pathophysiology of TIF [27]. Maladaptive growth factor (GF) activity and chronic inflammation seemingly initiate TIF, while subsequent oxidative stress constitutes a vicious microenvironment that fuels TIF progression. Peritubular capillary rarefaction and associated chronic hypoxia likely result from endothelial cell death under the biochemical/physical effect of matrix expansion and increased ROS production. Cell reprogramming is a (mal-)adaptive mechanism to the micro-environmental changes occurring in chronic diseases and cancers. To survive in this hypoxic and oxidative harmful environment, tubular cells undergo epithelial to mesenchymal transition (EMT) and accordingly, rewire their metabolic profile [28–30]. Cadherin switch or replacement of E-cadherin by N-cadherin is a key characteristic of EMT that reportedly plays an important role in the pathophysiology of TIF and can be reflective of the loss of renal parenchyma [31]. Considerable progress has been made in understanding the pathophysiology of TIF progression; however, the critical point of irreversibility in CKD progression remains a conundrum. Sustained GF/cytokine activity combined with an aberrant/excessive interstitial cell stimulation arguably constitutes a "self-enhancing loop" that promotes tubular injury and TIF. TGF-β is arguably the most potent profibrotic, though its effects depend upon the microenvironment, the dose, and the type of targeted cells. Mesenchymal activation of the Wnt/β-catenin pathway reportedly promotes fibrosis in experimental models of CKD. However, intact TGF-β/β-catenin activity is reportedly required to mediate PT adaptive response to chronic injury. TGF-β/β-catenin axis is therefore pivotal to studying post-injury PT regenerative capacity and the mechanisms leading to a maladaptive fibrotic response.

3. The kidney and proximal tubule (PT)

The kidney ensures body fluid and electrolytes homeostasis and secretes two hormones, renin and erythropoietin, respectively, regulating blood pressure and erythrocyte regeneration. Renal anatomy comprises two macroscopic parts: The cortex and the medulla. Its structural and functional unit, the nephron, includes the glomerulus and the tubular system. Under normal physiology, the kidney receives 20% of cardiac output (5 L/min), from which only 10% of the oxygen delivery is extracted. This inefficient use of oxygen in comparison to other metabolic organs such as the brain (34%) and the heart (65%) is due to the heterogeneous vascularization of the cortex and medulla. The bulk of renal blood flow (90%) is directed to the cortex (30 to 50 mmHg), resulting in a relatively low oxygen tension in the medulla (10 to 20 mmHg), creating a cortico-medullary metabolic switch [32–34]. The proximal tubule (PT), the most abundant segment dwelling in the renal cortex, relies on high cortical perfusion to achieve 70% water and sodium reabsorption and maintain its normal physiology [35, 36]. In end-stage renal disease (ESRD), the accumulation of extracellular matrix (ECM) proteins dramatically decreases cortical oxygen diffusion and imposes a metabolic adaptation in the PT to overcome chronic hypoxia and oxidative stress [37]. In addition to the cortico-medullary oxygen supply gradient, while distal renal epithelia express E-cadherin to ensure cell–cell adhesion, the PT relies on N-cadherin. N-cadherin is mostly expressed in mesenchymal cells and in high oxygen-dependent organs including the heart and the brain. Whether this E-to-N-cadherin switch plays a role in PT metabolism and survival in chronic injury is unknown. N-cadherin expression is targeted by TGF-β signaling, and its specific expression in the PT implies its possible role in PT oxidative metabolism. The PT is the most sensitive renal segment to injury partly due to its high metabolic rate and oxygen dependency but also its higher exposure to diverse toxins. PT energy supply relies on their abundant mitochondrial network, representing up to 40% of the PT cell volume, and the utilization of fatty acid beta-oxidation to couple oxygen consumption to ATP production [38–41]. The PT is divided into three parts: the convoluted tubules (S1 and S2) dwelling in the cortex and the parse recta (S3) located at the cortico-medullary junction and in the outer medulla (**Figure 1**). S3 PT cells are the most vulnerable to ischemia/toxins-induced acute kidney injury (AKI), and depending on the injury severity, injured cells dedifferentiate and proliferate or undergo necrosis [42, 43]. Mitochondria are crucial for PT cell survival by hosting and orchestrating intrinsic apoptosis. Injured PT is not only a victim but can become pivotal in the initiation of TIF progression through the paracrine effects of their secreted GFs and cytokines. Indeed, in acute kidney injury (AKI), injured PT cells

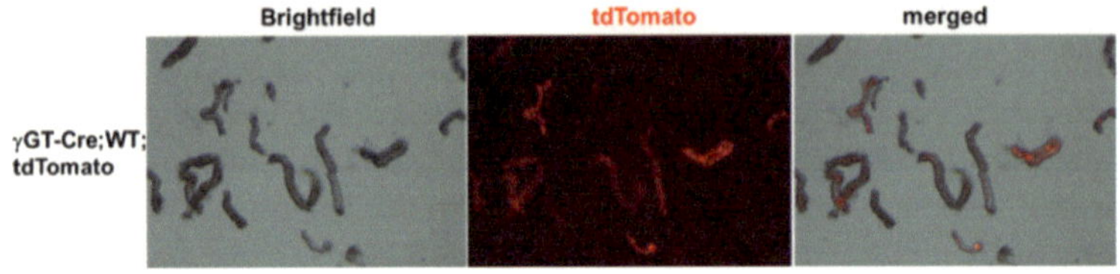

Figure 1.
Representative microscopy images of PTs (S3) isolated from tdTomato reporter mice carrying Cre-recombinase expression under the control of gamma-glutamyl transpeptidase (γGT-Cre; WT; tdTomato). From Dr. Nlandu Khodo Stellor.

secrete GFs and chemokines that promote epithelial recovery and reparative activation of interstitial cells, leading to post-injury recovery. However, in chronic injury, this tubulointerstitial crosstalk becomes maladaptive, leading to TIF [26, 44–47]. Thus, promoting adaptive PT cell response to chronic injury represents an important therapeutic strategy to counteract TIF progression. Among several pathways, TGF-β signaling has been reported to induce N-cadherin expression, a terminal differentiation marker of the PT cells [48], and Wnt/β-catenin is crucial in kidney development and β-catenin participates in the cellular structure integrity by linking cadherins to the actin cytoskeleton [49, 50].

4. TGF-β and β-catenin axis in tubule-interstitial fibrosis

4.1 TGF-β signaling

TGF-β is the most potent fibrotic factor in CKD. Three mammalian isoforms (TGF-β1, 2, and 3), encoded by distinct genes, have been identified. TGF-β1 is the predominant and best-characterized isoform and will be the focus of this chapter [51–53]. TGF-βs function through two serine/threonine kinase receptors, the type II (TbRII) and type I (TbRI or ALK5) TGF-β receptors. TβRII binds the active ligand and phosphorylates ALK5, which subsequently activates downstream Smad2/3. Active Smad2/3 oligomerizes with Smad4 and translocates to the nucleus, where their interactions with transcriptional co-factors lead to the expression of TGF-β target genes. TGF-β also activates Smad-independent pathways including MAP kinase [54, 55].

TGF-β signaling plays a pivotal role in normal (organ development, tissue homeostasis, and injury response) and pathological conditions (cancers and organ fibrosis) by mediating cell differentiation, migration, survival, and death. TGF-β signaling is required for kidney morphogenesis through inhibition of HGF-induced branching morphogenesis and promotion of tubule elongation [56, 57]. TGF-β displays multiple and opposing effects depending on the microenvironment and the targeted cell type. TGF-β is a tumor suppressor through induction of growth arrest and cell death; though it promotes malignancy by inducing epithelial to mesenchymal transition (EMT), particularly E-to-N-cadherin switch [58]. *TGF-β1* and *TbRII* knockout mice die around weaning age due to severe inflammation in most organ systems [59, 60]. Genetic or systemic/pharmacological inhibition of TGF-β mitigates TIF in mouse models of CKD; whereas kidney-specific Smad 2 knockout exacerbates TGF-β/Smad3 mediated fibrosis [61–63]. However, compelling data revealed the beneficial effect of the epithelial TGF-β signaling in experimental models of TIF, though the underlying subcellular mechanisms remained unclear in the last decades. Recent studies demonstrated that deletion of *TbRII* promotes PT cell survival and reduces TIF progression in two models of CKD by promoting cell survival and β-catenin activation, leading to reduced tubular injury (atrophy, dilatation, and flattening) and fibrosis (increased collagen accumulation) (**Figure 2**) [18]. Among multiple mechanisms in the pathophysiology of CKD, excessive TGF-β signaling has been reported to mediate mitochondria dysfunction through disruption of the electron transport chain (ETC) and suppression of antioxidant factors. However, TGF-β enhances mitochondrial function (oxygen consumption rate, mitochondrial membrane potential) and glycolysis in primary podocytes through activation of the mTOR pathway [64, 65]. Smad 2, a TGF-β's downstream effector, promotes mitochondrial fusion by interacting with mitofusin 2, a pro-fusion mitochondrial shaping protein. TGF-β induces autophagy/mitophagy, a protective mechanism whereby damaged organelles (mitochondria) are eliminated from cells and mediates mitochondrial elongation in ARPE-19 cells through the down-regulation of Opa3 [66–68]. TGF-β has been shown to induce the expression of glucose 6-phosphate dehydrogenase (G6pd), an enzyme that commits glucose breakdown to the pentose phosphate pathway. A recent study reported that TGF-β signaling mediates PT adaptive response to chronic injury by modulating mitochondrial homeostasis and Th1 immune response [69].

4.2 Wnt/β-catenin signaling

β-catenin is a multifunctional protein that functions as a structural anchor linking cell–cell adhesion proteins, notably cadherins, to the actin cytoskeleton at the adherens junctions. Interestingly, β-catenin is the signaling molecule of the Wnt/β-catenin pathway, which is crucial in organ development and in multiple pathogenic states including organ fibrosis and cancers. The binding of Wnts to the LRP/Frizzled receptor complex rescues β-catenin from phosphorylation by the destruction complex (Axin2/APC/GSK3β) and escapes the proteasomal degradation. This allows β-catenin cytosolic stabilization, nuclear translocation (activation), and interaction with its canonical co-transcriptional factors TCF/LEF to activate the transcription of pro-survival genes including c-myc, cyclin D1, and VEGF [70, 71]. β-catenin can also interact with other co-transcription factors, including FoxOs, to mediate non-canonical signaling [72].

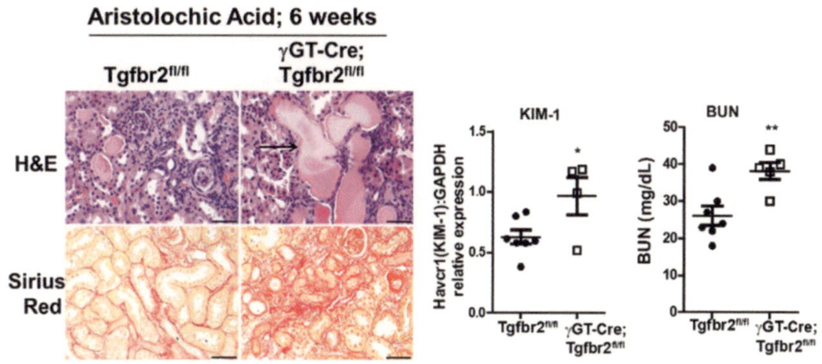

Figure 2.
H&E (structure), Sirius red (fibrosis) images showing deleterious (increased injury and fibrosis) effects of abrogating TGF-β signaling in mice lacking Tgfbr2 (TbRII) in the PT (γGT; Tgfbr2$^{fl/fl}$) upon aristolochic acid (AA)-induced CKD (left). Graphs showing increased PT injury (KIM-1) and decreased renal function as reflected by increased blood urea nitrogen (BUN) in AA-injured γGT;Tgfbr2$^{fl/fl}$ mice (from Nlandu Khodo et al. JASN 2017).

Wnt/β-catenin signaling mediates branching morphogenesis during kidney development. Wnt/β-catenin signaling is silenced in adult kidneys except in the inner medulla and is enhanced in both the cortex and medulla upon AKI to promote epithelial self-renewal potentially through reduction of apoptosis and/or altered proliferation [73–75]. Moreover, β-catenin and K-ras synergy leads to neoplasms, whereas its expression in the metanephric mesenchyme leads to renal dysplasia [76]. Wnt pathway is upregulated in biopsies of human diabetic kidneys and in PT of proteinuric human patients [22]. Several studies have shown the profibrotic effect of Wnt/β-catenin in fibroblasts/pericytes but not in renal epithelia. A study reported a maladaptive effect of Wnt signaling in the PT, but the authors overexpressed a Wnt ligand (Wnt9a), which likely had distant and maladaptive effects on interstitial/stromal cells [21]. Recent studies demonstrated the beneficial role of constitutive active β-catenin in PT under chronic tubular injury by reducing tubular injury and fibrosis (**Figure 3**) [25].

4.3 TGF-β/β-catenin axis and proximal tubule response to chronic injury

Sustained GFs/cytokines activity combined with aberrant/excessive interstitial cells stimulation arguably constitutes a "self-enhancing loop" that promotes tubular injury and TIF. Aberrant mesenchymal TGF-β and Wnt/β-catenin signaling arguably mediate TIF progression, though their effects depend on the type of targeted cells and the microenvironment. Experimental studies demonstrated that genetic inhibition of TGF-β signaling in the PT worsens TIF, and stabilization of β-catenin in the PT mitigates TIF under chronic injury, implying the pivotal role of synergistic β-catenin/TGF-β axis in PT adaptive response to chronic injury and survival [18, 25].

The TGF-β/β-catenin axis promotes cell differentiation, which is a prerequisite in post-injury survival prior to proliferation. Several studies illustrated the mechanisms whereby the TGF-β pathway activates Wnt/β-catenin signaling, though additional evidence must be provided to clarify how TGF-β regulates β-catenin activation in PT cells (**Figures 4–6**). According to the literature, TGF-β may regulate β-catenin activation at different levels of β-catenin signaling. TGF-β has been reported to inhibit DKK1, an inhibitor of the LRP5 receptor, suggesting a possible regulatory effect of TGF-β at the level of the receptor activation. TGF-β has been reported to promote

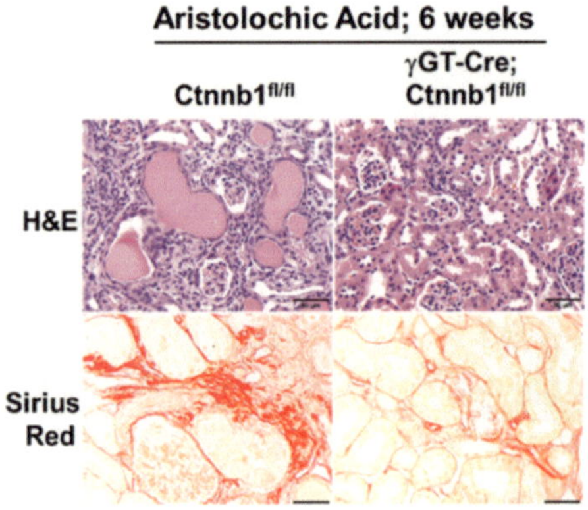

Figure 3.
H&E (structure) and Sirius red (fibrosis) images showing beneficial effects (decreased injury and fibrosis) in mice carrying constitutive stabilization of β-catenin in the PT (γGT;Ctnnb1$^{exo3fl/fl}$) upon AA-induced CKD (from Nlandu Khodo).

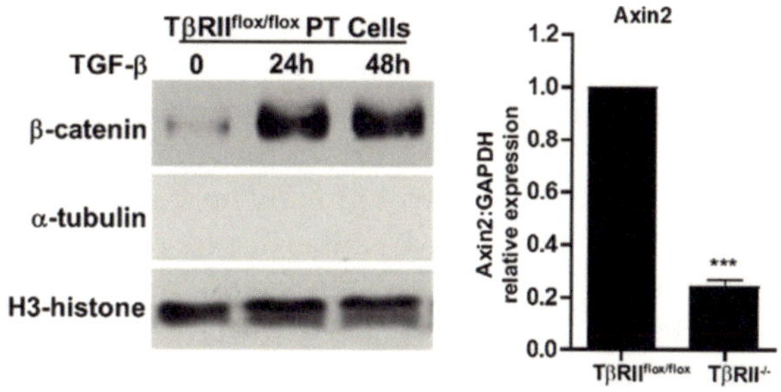

Figure 4.
Western blot showing increased β-catenin nuclear accumulation (activation) upon treatment of PT cells isolated from Tgfbr2$^{fl/fl}$ *mice (TβRII*$^{flox/flox}$*) with TGF-β. α-tubulin and H3-histone are used as cytosolic and nuclear fraction markers, respectively (left). qPCR showing basal decrease of canonical β-catenin transcriptional activity as reflected by decreased Axin2 in PT cells lacking TbRII (TβRII*$^{-/-}$*) (from Nlandu Khodo et al. JASN 2017).*

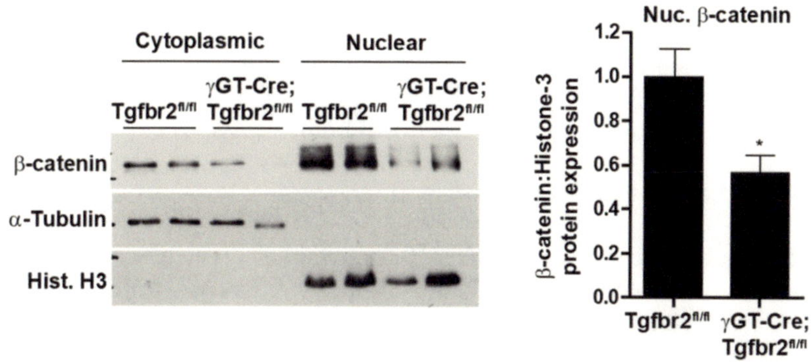

Figure 5.
Western blot and quantification showing decreased β-catenin nuclear accumulation (activation) in mice lacking Tgfbr2 (TbRII) in the PT (γGT;Tgfbr2$^{fl/fl}$*) 3 weeks after AA-induced injury. α-tubulin and H3-histone are used as cytosolic and nuclear fraction markers, respectively (from Nlandu Khodo et al. JASN 2017).*

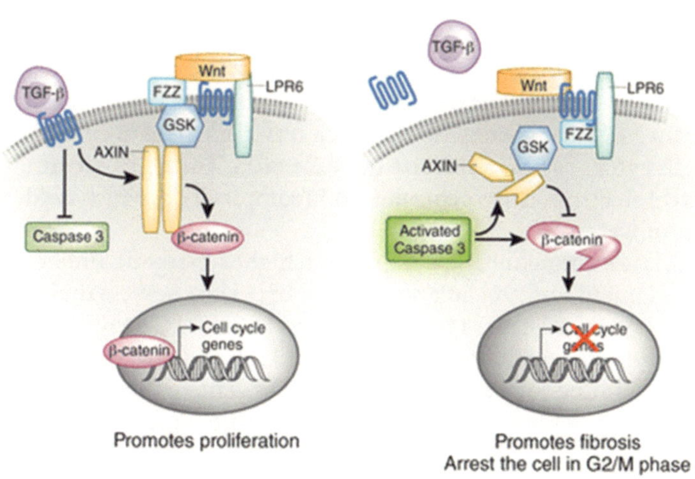

Figure 6.
TGF-β receptor signaling is proposed to facilitate successful recovery from cellular damage by interacting with the Wnt-β-catenin pathway. Genetic ablation of the TGF-β receptor in proximal tubule inhibits normal nuclear localization of β-catenin, resulting in increased death, cell cycle arrest, and expression of fibrotic factors (from Basile DP and Mehrotra P, JASN 2017).

Ser9 phosphorylation of GSK3β, leading to its inactivation and, subsequently, to β-catenin activation; finally, several studies have reported a direct interaction of pSMAD3 and with β-catenin that prevents β-catenin degradation and promotes its nuclear accumulation [77–79]. β-Catenin is one of the components of the intercellular junctions (aderens junctions), where it directly interacts with the intracellular fragments of cadherins. TGF-β represses E-cadherin expression while increasing N-cadherin expression [80, 81]. The TGF-β's repressive effect on E-cadherin expression involves the activation of zinc-finger transcription factors including Snail1, Slug, and Twist1. Recent studies in human PT cells (HK-2) reported the role of histone deacetylase (Hdac), particularly Hdac8, as an important regulator of TGF-β repressive effect on E-cadherin expression. Moreover, TGF-β may post-transcriptionally regulate cadherin expression through the induction of proteinases including Sheddases (ADAM 10 and TACE) and other metalloproteases [82]. This repressive effect of TGF-β signaling on E-cadherin may increase β-catenin cytosolic pool and promote its activation. Decreased E-cadherin expression has been reported to increase β-catenin cytosolic pool and promote β-catenin signaling [83]. TGF-β signaling induces N-cadherin expression in PT cells, and the putative expression of N-cadherin in the PT implies an intrinsic role of TGF-β signaling in the maintenance of PT cell terminal differentiation and functional homeostasis.

4.3.1 TGF-β/β-catenin axis and mitochondria

Mitochondria are cylindrical organelles (0.5 to 1 mm of diameter) delimited by a double membrane, outer (OMM) and inner (IMM) membranes, which form two compartments: inter-membrane space (IMS) and mitochondrial matrix. The OMM is less specialized and quasi-permeable to small molecules compared to the IMM, which is selectively permeable and forms a series of folds (cristae) projecting into the matrix. The matrix is the site of the tricarboxylic acid cycle (TCA), which performs the oxidation of Acetyl-CoA from multiple sources (hexoses, fatty and amino acids) to generate NADH, further converted to adenosine-5′-triphosphate (ATP), through the IMM electron transport chain (ETC). The ETC is composed of four multi-protein complexes that receive and transfer electrons and create a proton (H+) gradient to generate ATP using F0F1 ATPase (complex V) enzymatic activity. The NADH coenzyme Q reductase or NADH dehydrogenase (complex I) accepts and transfers 2 electrons from NADH to coenzyme Q, which transfers them to cytochrome bc1 or coenzyme QH2-cytochrome c reductase (complex III). Through cytochrome c, complex III transfers electrons to cytochrome AA3 (complex IV), which reduces oxygen in two molecules of water.

Mitochondria are abundant and elongated in highly energetic and healthier cells, whereas they fragment under cellular stress [84, 85]. They possess their own genome of 16.6 K bp, coding for 37 genes (13 polypeptides of the ETC enzymes, 22 tRNA, and 2 rRNA); however, most mitochondrial proteins (1100) involved in mDNA replication, structure, and function come from the nuclear genome, implying a considerable role of nuclear genome derived factors in the maintenance of mitochondria homeostasis.

The mechanism whereby TGF-β signaling affects ETC protein expression and function remains unclear for a long time. Mitochondria are composed of proteins coded by their own genome and nuclear genome, and mitochondrial protein sorting and localization are tightly regulated. Nuclear genome-coded protein import into mitochondria is mediated by different translocases and porins. The Tomm complex and Vdac (in the OMM) are involved in protein import into the IMS while Timm23/Pam3 (in the IMM) complex facilitates their transport to the mitochondrial matrix. The sorting and assembly machinery (SAM) and Timm22 are involved in protein insertion into the OMM and IMM, respectively [86, 87]. Mitochondria are the cornerstone of PT cell metabolism and survival, respectively, through fatty acid oxidation (FAO) and modulation of response to apoptosis/injury. They represent an important proportion of PT cell volume while cells of the inner medulla, displaying parsimonious oxygen consumption, have lower mitochondrial density. Given its high dependency on mitochondrial oxygen metabolism, the PT necessitates a powerful antioxidant buffering system to neutralize mitochondrial metabolism-derived ROS and maintain its functional integrity.

The quality control of mitochondria is regulated at different levels: morphology, density, and function. The morphology is mainly regulated by mitochondrial shaping proteins (MSP), which mainly include pro-fission (dynamin-related protein Drp1 and its downstream Fis1), pro-fusion (Mfn1/2 and the dynamin family GTPase Opa1) proteins. Several studies have reported the pivotal role of Pgc-1α in mitochondrial biogenesis, while Pink1/Parkin and BNIP3/Nix have been associated with cell disposal of damaged mitochondria through mitophagy [88, 89]. Mitochondrial dysfunction has been implicated in a broad range of inherited and acquired renal diseases, including tubular defects (Fanconi and Bartter-like syndromes), cystic disease, AKI, glomerular diseases (FSGS), and CKD. Several data have reported disruption of mitochondrial respiration in TIF, including inactivation of complex IV in CKD patients [90]. The uremic toxins impair ETC function and cause cell dedifferentiation. Moreover, the reduction of mitochondrial copy number and increased oxidative stress in skeletal muscle is associated with CKD in humans and mice [91].

TGF-β signaling is necessary to maintain and promote homeostatic OXPHOS, and excessive TGF-β signaling has detrimental effects on oxygen consumption rate (OCR) and ATP production. PT cells lacking *TbRII* show decreased basal OCR and slightly increased extracellular acidification rate (ECAR) in line with decreased mitochondrial coupling efficiency, suggesting that TGF-β signaling inhibition directly impacts the PT cell's capacity to efficiently produce ATP via OXPHOS. The absence of TGF-β signaling in mouse PT cells induces a metabolic switch from OXPHOS to increased lactate production consistent with anaerobic glycolysis preference and decreased expression of the polymerase γ. Moreover, the ubiquinone metabolism and complex I are the most affected pathway in PT cells lacking the *TbRII*, implying that deletion of *TbRII* induces mitochondrial dysfunction and metabolic switch, partly through impaired expression and function of complex I subunits. Mitochondria homeostasis involves its quality control, which is mainly mediated by their renewal through biogenesis and mitophagy. Pgc1α, the master regulator of mitochondrial biogenesis, has been shown to protect against CKD, though it is regulated in a dose-dependent manner by TGF-β. PT cells lacking the *TbRII* have decreased Pink1 protein level, an important protein in mitophagy, suggesting that TGF-β signaling regulates mitochondrial homeostasis by promoting mitophagy and expression of complex I subunits [69].

4.3.2 TGF-β/β-catenin axis and inflammation

TGF-β is a multi-faceted cytokine that mediates pro-and anti-inflammatory responses depending on the microenvironment and the targeted cell types. However, global *TbRII* or TGF-β1 knockout causes lethal inflammatory disorders in mice, notably by regulating lymphocyte homeostasis [59, 60], suggesting its intrinsic anti-inflammatory function. Mitochondrial damage-associated molecular patterns (DAMPS) reportedly lead to the activation of Cgas/Sting/IFNγ axis in renal fibrosis [92, 93]. Though macrophages and dendritic cells initiate inflammation in response to tubular injury, T cells are involved in the whole evolution of injury [94]. Abrogation of TGF-β signaling in the PT leads to increased IFNγ and TNFα+ CD4+ cells in kidneys, whereas CD8+ cells are augmented but not significantly different between genotypes. Moreover, the percentage of the reno-protective Foxp3+ (T reg) CD4+ cells out of CD45+ cells is decreased in the kidneys of mice lacking *TbRII* in the PT cells. Cgas/Sting proteins, which are responsive to DAMPS and induction of IFNγ, are reportedly increased in the absence of *TbRII* in the PT, suggesting that *TbRII* deletion-induced mitochondrial dysfunction worsens Th1 inflammatory response in acute to chronic PT injury models in mice [69]. Consistently, several studies reported the anti-inflammatory effect of Wnt/β-catenin activation by inhibiting TNFα and IFNγ pathways [95–97]. Taken together, PT specific TGF-β/β-catenin axis activation ameliorates response to chronic injury, partly, by promoting expression of epithelial factors that mediate renal recovery ("PRLs") which can act autonomously at the level of PT metabolism (mitochondria) and inflammatory cell–cell communication (**Figure 7**).

4.3.3 TGF-β/β-catenin axis and cell cycle

The cell cycle is a ubiquitous and highly coordinated process involved in organ development and tissue homeostasis whose dysfunctions lead to several pathological

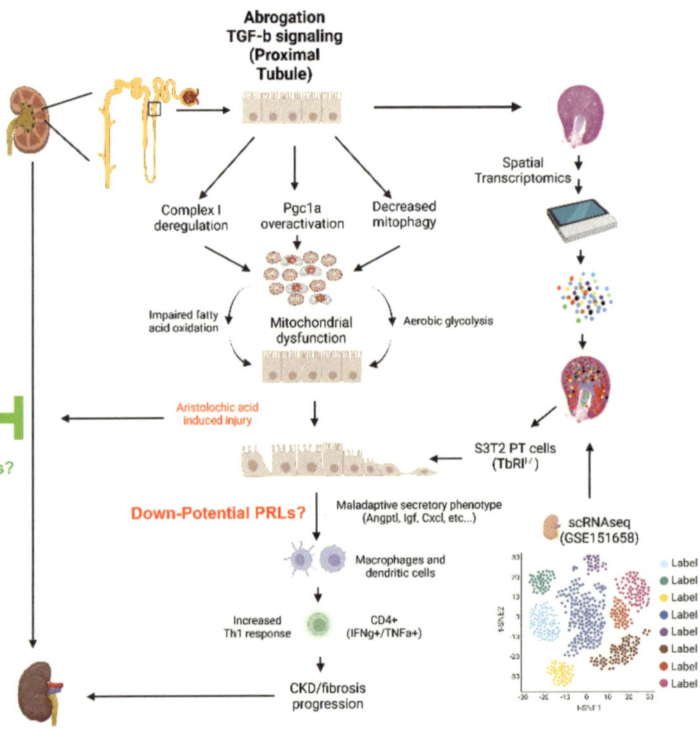

Figure 7.
Illustration depicting the mechanisms whereby abrogation of TGF-β signaling worsens chronic kidney disease (CKD)/TIF (Nlandu Khodo S et al. JASN 2017; Kayhan M et al. Nat. Comm 2023).

states including CKD [98]. It is characterized by the phase of nuclear division (mitosis) and the interlude between two mitoses (interphase). The mitosis (M phase) is divided into four stages (prophase, metaphase, anaphase, and telophase) characterized by chromosomal dynamics and segregation into two daughter nuclei. The interphase is composed of the G1, S, and G2 phases. The S phase is characterized by DNA replication while G1 and G2 phases are cell cycle gaps during which the cell is prepared for DNA synthesis and mitosis, respectively.

The cell cycle arrest is an important mechanism during kidney injury response whose dysfunction participates in the pathogenesis of CKD. While G0/G1 cell cycle arrest is considered as a mechanism contributing to the maintenance of organ homeostasis, G2/M cell cycle arrest has been associated with the maladaptive repair process following kidney injury and increased susceptibility to cell death. The G1 phase of the cell cycle is an intermediate stable state during which the two daughter cells that exit the mitosis must sense and integrate the microenvironmental stimuli to enter a resting stage (G0) or to, commit to a new cycle or die.

The cell cycle integrity is intimately regulated by cyclin-dependent kinases (CDKs), a family of serine/threonine protein kinases activated at specific points of the cell cycle. CDK activation necessitates interaction with proteins called cyclins, whose expressions fluctuate throughout the cell cycle, ensuring periodic and specific activation of CDKs during the cell cycle. Several studies identified specific CDK/Cyclin interactions during the progression of the cell cycle, notably in G1 (CDK2, CDK4, CDK6 and Cyclins type D/E), S (CDK2 and cyclin type A), G2 and M (CDK1 and Cyclins type A/B). The G1/S phase transition is characterized by the retinoblastoma protein (Rb) hyperphosphorylation and activation of E2F transcription factors, and these two events constitute the restriction point (R point) or the commitment to a new cell cycle. In addition to CDK/Cyclins, the cell cycle is also controlled by two families of Cyclin-dependent kinase inhibitors (CKIs), the INK4 (p15, p16, p18, and p19) and the Cip/Kip (p21, p27, and p57). CKIs counteract the cell cycle progression by specifically binding to CKDs or CKD/Cyclin complexes. The INK4 family specifically inactivates G1 CDK (CDK4 and CDK6) while the Cip/Kip family inhibits G1 CDK/Cyclins complexes and M CDK/Cyclin complex (CDK1/Cyclin type B).

Activation of TGF-β, known for its role in organ development and tissue homeostasis, has been reported to regulate both G2/M and G1 cell cycle arrest in dose and context-dependent manner. This effect may be inherent to the pleiotropic nature of TGF-β signaling or likely mediated by some of its downstream effectors, such as Forkhead box O 1 (FoxO1) transcription factor, known to induce G1 arrest and mediate cytoprotection under oxidative stress. Depending on the dose, TGF-β-induces cell cycle arrest at G0/G1 or G2/M phases [99–101]. TGF-β-induced cell cycle arrest at G0/G1 is likely the mechanism by which this growth factor promotes survival in chronic kidney injury. Indeed, though renal epithelia are relatively quiescent in homeostasis, renal injury stimulates cell cycle entry. Most compelling data demonstrate that epithelial cells in either G0 or G1 have improved survival in response to chronic stress (oxidative stress, hypoxia, toxins, ...) than cells at later stages in the cell cycle (S, G2/M), which are more vulnerable to apoptosis [102, 103]. TGF-β stimulates G1 arrest in epithelial cells, likely through multiple pathways that target CDK, which, in conjunction with cyclins, promote G1 progression to S [104–106]. Two families of CDK inhibitors that play an important role in regulating TGF-β-dependent G1 arrest are INK4 and the Cip/Kip family [107–110]. G1 arrest may also be beneficial by decreasing the number of injured epithelia that progress to G2 arrest. Other authors have shown that injured renal epithelia that are arrested in G2/M acquire a secretory phenotype and produce increased amounts of profibrotic GFs in chronic renal injury [111]. Palbociclib, recently FDA-approved for breast cancer, induces G1 arrest by inhibiting CDK4/6, a mechanism like that of the INK4 family of CDK inhibitors. This pharmacologic inhibitor protected renal function in a murine model of acute kidney injury and CKD [112]. TGF-β signaling in renal epithelia increases transcription of INK4 proteins (e.g., p15INK4B) but not that of Cip/Kip family members p21 or p27. Consistent with an inhibition of CDK4/6, TGF-β signaling increases the number of PT cells in G0/G1 and reduces G2/M arrest. By inducing G1 arrest, TGF-β signaling may augment epithelial cell survival in the hypoxic CKD microenvironment and decrease TIF by limiting the number of epithelial cells that progress to G2/M arrest [113]. FoxO1, a forkhead transcription factor and established regulator of G1 arrest, is regulated by TGF-β signaling in mouse PT cells [114]. TGF-β and FoxO1 promote G1 arrest in a variety of ways, but they both target similar CDK inhibitors of the INK4 and Cip/Kip families. In fact, FoxO has been reported to interact with Smads and promote transcription of the p15INK4B gene, a well-described target of TGF-β [115, 116]. TGF-β may augment FoxO1-mediated G1 arrest through both increased FoxO1 transcription and through interactions with Smads to promote the expression of CDK inhibitors [115, 117, 118]. Treatment of PT cells with BIO, a β-catenin activator, decreases aristolochic acid toxicity-induced G2/M arrest and promotes G0/G1 arrest in the absence of TGF-β signaling in accordance with the synergistic interaction between TGF-β and β-catenin in cell cycle regulation in PT cells [18].

5. Discussion

CKD is a silent-onset disease mainly caused by diabetes and hypertension. Regardless of the initial insult, tubulointerstitial fibrosis (TIF) is the hallmark of late-stage CKD that directly correlates with the loss of renal function. Though our understanding of the pathophysiology of CKD has tremendously improved in the last decades, there is no curative treatment for CKD patients. Alternative replacement therapies include dialysis and renal transplantation. Renal injury can occur at both the glomerular and the tubulointerstitial (lesions in the renal tubules/proximal tubules and the peritubular capillaries) compartments, leading to elevated level of proteins in the urine (proteinuria) and the decline of the glomerular filtration rate (GFR). The treatments are adjusted according to the disease etiology and target the amelioration of specific clinical parameters, notably proteinuria and GFR. Several mechanisms intertwine in the pathophysiology of CKD, including chronic hypoxia, inflammation, oxidative stress, and cell reprogramming, and have been targeted to mitigate CKD progression in animals and patients [119–121]. The activation of the renin-angiotensin-aldosterone (RAA) system in response to injury-induced systemic and intrarenal hemodynamic changes is a common pathophysiological feature that fuels CKD progression. Thus, RAAS inhibitors and voltage-dependent calcium channel antagonists have been the main therapeutic strategies to slow CKD progression, and specific families of these inhibitors/antagonists are adjusted according to the patient's history [122]. Renal anemia is an important feature of CKD progression, which is traditionally treated by recombinant erythropoietin (Epo) supplementation. The elucidation of the molecular principles of oxygen-sensing which control Epo production, notably the HIF-PHD-VHL interplay, in the last few years (Nobel Prize 2019) has led to the development of novel oral PHD inhibitors as a potential alternative to the expensive Epo supplementation to treat anemic CKD patients, though a better understanding of the renal oxygen-signaling pathway becomes even more crucial

[123]. Lately, sodium-glucose transport protein 2 (SGLT2) inhibitors have emerged as an efficient strategy to treat CKD patients while providing cardiovascular benefits [124, 125]. TGF-β is a pleiotropic factor and arguably the most potent profibrotic factor in CKD progression. TGF-β and Wnt/β-catenin axis is emerging as an important pathway that couples renal epithelial homeostasis and oxygen metabolism. TGF-β signaling interferes with most of the therapeutic targets in CKD treatment including the RAA system and HIF pathway [126–129]. Upon chronic injury, growth factors including TGF-β and Wnt/β-catenin orchestrate tubulointerstitial interactions, which lead to stromal/interstitial cell activation and fibrosis. Although several studies have demonstrated the harmful effects of systemic TGF-β activation, targeted TGF-β signaling inhibition has not revealed beneficial in clinical studies. Previous study demonstrated that pan-mesenchymal inhibition of TGF-β signaling does not mitigate CKD progression [15]. Surprisingly, a recent study has shown that deletion of Tgfbr2 in Pdgfrβ positive cells prevents the decline of Epo production without altering fibrosis [130]. However, by targeting a broad population of stromal cells, it is difficult to sort out the intrinsic effect of TGF-β signaling on renal erythropoietic cells from the effect of cellular interaction within the subpopulation. Abrogation of TGF-β signaling in the proximal tubule (PT), the most vulnerable renal segment to injury, worsens CKD in mice [18, 69]. TGF-β signaling reportedly induces G1 cell cycle arrest; pharmacological induction of G1/S cell cycle arrest using selective inhibitor of CDK4/6 revealed protection in mouse models of CKD [113]. As TGF-β signaling, Wnt/β-catenin signaling displays multiple and opposing effects in renal fibrosis. While mesenchymal activation of Wnt/β-catenin promotes renal fibrosis, its proximal tubular activation mitigates CKD progression partly by activating cytoprotective/antioxidant pathways [25]. Despite its beneficial effect in PT response to injury, long-term activation of Wnt/β-catenin leads to neoplasms and increase the risk of developing renal tumors in case of activating K-RAS mutation [76].

Given the current findings and the pleiotropic effects (cell type, microenvironment, and dose dependency) of TGF-β and Wnt/β-catenin axis, it will be difficult to systemically target these pathways as therapeutics strategies to treat CKD patients due to potential on and off-target side effects. Nanoparticle drug delivery strategies (DDS) can be used to specifically target TGF-β and Wnt/β-catenin activation in specific cell types, notably in PT cells, and overcome the deleterious effect of systemic activation of TGF-β and Wnt/β-catenin axis in clinical studies. Though the proposed approach appears promising, future studies should aim to identify downstream effectors whereby the TGF-β and Wnt/β-catenin axis mediate PT adaptive response to chronic renal injury.

6. Conclusion

Chronic kidney disease (CKD) is a growing health problem affecting 10% of the global population, and this number will likely increase given the huge burden of diabetes and hypertension, the two leading causes of CKD. Glomerular and tubulointerstitial injuries both lead to CKD through progressive tubulointerstitial fibrosis (TIF), and chronic tubular injury is an important component in the pathophysiology of TIF progression. Understanding how tubular epithelia respond to chronic injury is therefore crucial for the development of effective therapy to halt CKD progression. TGF-β is uncontestable, the master profibrotic factor involved in the pathophysiology of CKD, and Wnt/β-catenin activation in mesenchymal cells promotes renal fibrosis. However, these two pathways mediate many different responses, some of which may be beneficial in renal chronic injury.

This chapter summarizes the most recent findings describing the mechanisms whereby the TGF-β/β-catenin axis mediates proximal tubule (PT) adaptive response to chronic renal injury. TGF-β/β-catenin axis mediates PT adaptive response to chronic injury by promoting mitochondrial homeostasis, adaptive Th1 inflammatory response, and promotes G0/G1 cell cycle arrest upon chronic renal injury. Several mechanisms can be targeted to hamper CKD progression including complex I expression and function, oxidative stress, glycolysis, mitophagy, Th1 immune response, and cell cycle arrest. Targeting inhibition of the TGF-β/β-catenin axis failed to mitigate CKD in clinical practice. Although promoting tubular TGF-β/β-catenin axis signaling revealed benefits upon chronic injury in mice, it is not safe to pharmacologically target direct TGF-β/β-catenin activation as a therapeutic strategy against CKD due to its pleiotropic effects. However, identification of post-injury key regenerative effectors in this axis may help to pinpoint specific anti-fibrotic factors that can be targeted to mitigate CKD progression in humans.

Acknowledgements

I acknowledge Professor Leslie Gewin for directing the project on the role of TGF-β signaling and β-catenin in the proximal tubule response to chronic injury at Vanderbilt University Medical Center and for her tremendous mentoring contribution to my career; and Professor Roland Wenger for hosting my research group in the Institute of Physiology, Faculties of Medicine and Sciences, University of Zurich.

This work was supported by the Swiss National Science Foundation (AMBIZIONE grant PZ00P3_179916 and the NCCR "Kidney.CH" junior grant to S.N.K.).

Conflict of interest

The author has no conflicts of interest.

Author details

Stellor Nlandu Khodo
Faculty of Medicine and Sciences, Institute of Physiology, University of Zurich, Zurich, Switzerland

*Address all correspondence to: stellor.nlandukhodo@uzh.ch

References

[1] Friedman SL et al. Therapy for fibrotic diseases: Nearing the starting line. Science Translational Medicine. 2013;**5**(167):167sr1

[2] Rosenbloom J, Castro SV, Jimenez SA. Narrative review: Fibrotic diseases: Cellular and molecular mechanisms and novel therapies. Annals of Internal Medicine. 2010;**152**(3):159-166

[3] Voelker J et al. Anti-TGF-beta1 antibody therapy in patients with diabetic nephropathy. Journal of the American Society of Nephrology. 2017;**28**(3):953-962

[4] Amann K, Tyralla K. Cardiovascular changes in chronic renal failure–pathogenesis and therapy. Clinical Nephrology. 2002;**58**(Suppl. 1):S62-S72

[5] Bohle A et al. The pathogenesis of chronic renal failure. Pathology, Research and Practice. 1989;**185**(4):421-440

[6] Isbel NM et al. Increased targeting of cardiovascular risk factors in patients with chronic kidney disease does not improve atheroma burden or cardiovascular function. American Heart Journal. 2006;**151**(3):745-753

[7] McMurray JJ et al. Predictors of fatal and nonfatal cardiovascular events in patients with type 2 diabetes mellitus, chronic kidney disease, and anemia: An analysis of the trial to reduce cardiovascular events with Aranesp (darbepoetin-alfa) therapy (TREAT). American Heart Journal. 2011;**162**(4):748-755 e3

[8] Parikh NI et al. Cardiovascular disease risk factors in chronic kidney disease: Overall burden and rates of treatment and control. Archives of Internal Medicine. 2006;**166**(17):1884-1891

[9] Pergola PE et al. Economic burden and health-related quality of life associated with current treatments for anaemia in patients with CKD not on dialysis: A systematic review. PharmacoEconomics - Open. 2019

[10] Thorp ML et al. Managing the burden of chronic kidney disease. Disease Management. 2006;**9**(2): 115-121

[11] Vanholder R et al. Reducing the costs of chronic kidney disease while delivering quality health care: A call to action. Nature Reviews. Nephrology. 2017;**13**(7):393-409

[12] Meng XM, Nikolic-Paterson DJ, Lan HY. TGF-beta: The master regulator of fibrosis. Nature Reviews. Nephrology. 2016;**12**(6):325-338

[13] Tan RJ et al. Wnt/beta-catenin signaling and kidney fibrosis. Kidney International Supplements (2011). 2014;**4**(1):84-90

[14] Gewin L et al. TGF-beta receptor deletion in the renal collecting system exacerbates fibrosis. Journal of the American Society of Nephrology. 2010;**21**(8):1334-1343

[15] Neelisetty S et al. Renal fibrosis is not reduced by blocking transforming growth factor-beta signaling in matrix-producing interstitial cells. Kidney International. 2015;**88**(3):503-514

[16] Derynck R et al. An emerging complexity of receptors for transforming growth factor-beta. Princess Takamatsu Symposia. 1994;**24**:264-275

[17] Kubiczkova L et al. TGF-beta - An excellent servant but a bad master. Journal of Translational Medicine. 2012;**10**:183

[18] Nlandu-Khodo S et al. Blocking TGF-beta and beta-catenin epithelial crosstalk exacerbates CKD. Journal of the American Society of Nephrology. 2017;**28**(12):3490-3503

[19] Wakefield LM, Roberts AB. TGF-beta signaling: Positive and negative effects on tumorigenesis. Current Opinion in Genetics & Development. 2002;**12**(1):22-29

[20] Kramann R et al. Matrix producing cells in chronic kidney disease: Origin, regulation, and activation. Current Pathobiology Reports. 2013;**1**(4)

[21] Luo C et al. Wnt9a promotes renal fibrosis by accelerating cellular senescence in tubular epithelial cells. Journal of the American Society of Nephrology. 2018;**29**(4):1238-1256

[22] Rudnicki M et al. Gene expression profiles of human proximal tubular epithelial cells in proteinuric nephropathies. Kidney International. 2007;**71**(4):325-335

[23] Zhou D et al. Wnt/beta-catenin signaling in kidney injury and repair: A double-edged sword. Laboratory Investigation. 2016;**96**(2):156-167

[24] Zhou D et al. Kidney tubular beta-catenin signaling controls interstitial fibroblast fate via epithelial-mesenchymal communication. Scientific Reports. 2013;**3**:1878

[25] Nlandu-Khodo S et al. Tubular beta-catenin and FoxO3 interactions protect in chronic kidney disease. JCI Insight. 2020;**5**(10)

[26] Bonventre JV, Yang L. Cellular pathophysiology of ischemic acute kidney injury. The Journal of Clinical Investigation. 2011;**121**(11):4210-4221

[27] Matovinovic MS. 1. Pathophysiology and classification of kidney diseases. EJIFCC. 2009;**20**(1):2-11

[28] Kang H et al. Role of metabolic reprogramming in epithelial(−) mesenchymal transition (EMT). International Journal of Molecular Sciences. 2019;**20**(8)

[29] Rosland GV et al. Epithelial to mesenchymal transition (EMT) is associated with attenuation of succinate dehydrogenase (SDH) in breast cancer through reduced expression of SDHC. Cancer & Metabolism. 2019;**7**:6

[30] Sciacovelli M, Frezza C. Metabolic reprogramming and epithelial-to-mesenchymal transition in cancer. The FEBS Journal. 2017;**284**(19):3132-3144

[31] Nlandu Khodo S et al. NADPH-oxidase 4 protects against kidney fibrosis during chronic renal injury. Journal of the American Society of Nephrology. 2012;**23**(12):1967-1976

[32] Brezis M, Rosen S. Hypoxia of the renal medulla--its implications for disease. The New England Journal of Medicine. 1995;**332**(10):647-655

[33] Epstein FH. Oxygen and renal metabolism. Kidney International. 1997;**51**(2):381-385

[34] Heyman SN, Fuchs S, Brezis M. The role of medullary ischemia in acute renal failure. New Horizons. 1995;**3**(4):597-607

[35] Giebisch G. Kidney, water and electrolyte metabolism. Annual Review of Physiology. 1962;**24**:357-420

[36] Whittembury G et al. Some aspects of proximal tubular sodium chloride reabsorption in Necturus kidney. Kidney International. 1975;**7**(5):293-230

[37] Mimura I, Nangaku M. The suffocating kidney: Tubulointerstitial hypoxia in end-stage renal disease. Nature Reviews. Nephrology. 2010;**6**(11):667-678

[38] Chevalier RL. The proximal tubule is the primary target of injury and progression of kidney disease: Role of the glomerulotubular junction. American Journal of Physiology. Renal Physiology. 2016;**311**(1):F145-F161

[39] Forbes MS et al. A population of mitochondrion-rich cells in the pars recta of mouse kidney. Cell and Tissue Research. 2016;**363**(3):791-803

[40] Silva P. Renal fuel utilization, energy requirements, and function. Kidney International. Supplement. 1987;**22**:S9-S14

[41] Suzuki T et al. Giant mitochondria in the epithelial cells of the proximal convoluted tubules of diseased human kidneys. Laboratory Investigation. 1975;**33**(6):578-590

[42] Liu BC et al. Renal tubule injury: A driving force toward chronic kidney disease. Kidney International. 2018;**93**(3):568-579

[43] Qi R, Yang C. Renal tubular epithelial cells: The neglected mediator of tubulointerstitial fibrosis after injury. Cell Death & Disease. 2018;**9**(11):1126

[44] Begnaud S et al. Mechanics of epithelial tissues during gap closure. Current Opinion in Cell Biology. 2016;**42**:52-62

[45] Castrop H. The role of renal interstitial cells in proximal tubular regeneration. Nephron. 2019;**141**(4):265-272

[46] Chen J et al. Survivin mediates renal proximal tubule recovery from AKI. Journal of the American Society of Nephrology. 2013;**24**(12):2023-2033

[47] Zhang Y et al. GDF11 improves tubular regeneration after acute kidney injury in elderly mice. Scientific Reports. 2016;**6**:34624

[48] Keller C et al. Distinct mesenchymal alterations in N-cadherin and E-cadherin positive primary renal epithelial cells. PLoS One. 2012;**7**(8):e43584

[49] Boivin FJ et al. The good and bad of beta-catenin in kidney development and renal dysplasia. Frontiers in Cell and Development Biology. 2015;**3**:81

[50] Deacon P et al. Beta-catenin regulates the formation of multiple nephron segments in the mouse kidney. Scientific Reports. 2019;**9**(1):15915

[51] Lawrence DA. Transforming growth factor-beta: A general review. European Cytokine Network. 1996;**7**(3):363-374

[52] Mourskaia AA et al. Transforming growth factor-beta1 is the predominant isoform required for breast cancer cell outgrowth in bone. Oncogene. 2009;**28**(7):1005-1015

[53] Yu L et al. TGF-beta isoforms in renal fibrogenesis. Kidney International. 2003;**64**(3):844-856

[54] Derynck R, Zhang YE. Smad-dependent and Smad-independent pathways in TGF-beta family signalling. Nature. 2003;**425**(6958):577-584

[55] Massague J. TGF-beta signal transduction. Annual Review of Biochemistry. 1998;**67**:753-791

[56] Massague J. TGF-beta signaling in development and disease. FEBS Letters. 2012;**586**(14):1833

[57] Oxburgh L et al. TGFbeta superfamily signals are required for morphogenesis of the kidney mesenchyme progenitor population. Development. 2004;**131**(18):4593-4605

[58] Bachman KE, Park BH. Duel nature of TGF-beta signaling: Tumor suppressor vs. tumor promoter. Current Opinion in Oncology. 2005;**17**(1):49-54

[59] Bommireddy R et al. TGF-beta 1 regulates lymphocyte homeostasis by preventing activation and subsequent apoptosis of peripheral lymphocytes. Journal of Immunology. 2003;**170**(9):4612-4622

[60] Leveen P et al. Induced disruption of the transforming growth factor beta type II receptor gene in mice causes a lethal inflammatory disorder that is transplantable. Blood. 2002;**100**(2):560-568

[61] Inazaki K et al. Smad3 deficiency attenuates renal fibrosis, inflammation,and apoptosis after unilateral ureteral obstruction. Kidney International. 2004;**66**(2):597-604

[62] Kellenberger T et al. Differential effects of Smad3 targeting in a murine model of chronic kidney disease. Physiological Reports. 2013;**1**(7):e00181

[63] Meng XM et al. Smad2 protects against TGF-beta/Smad3-mediated renal fibrosis. Journal of the American Society of Nephrology. 2010;**21**(9):1477-1487

[64] Abe Y et al. TGF-beta1 stimulates mitochondrial oxidative phosphorylation and generation of reactive oxygen species in cultured mouse podocytes, mediated in part by the mTOR pathway. American Journal of Physiology. Renal Physiology. 2013;**305**(10):F1477-F1490

[65] Yoon YS et al. TGF beta1 induces prolonged mitochondrial ROS generation through decreased complex IV activity with senescent arrest in Mv1Lu cells. Oncogene. 2005;**24**(11):1895-1903

[66] Heine UI et al. Localization of transforming growth factor-beta 1 in mitochondria of murine heart and liver. Cell Regulation. 1991;**2**(6):467-477

[67] Ryu SW et al. Downregulation of OPA3 is responsible for transforming growth factor-beta-induced mitochondrial elongation and F-actin rearrangement in retinal pigment epithelial ARPE-19 cells. PLoS One. 2013;**8**(5):e63495

[68] Shah N, Lee NY. Regulation of gene expression and mitochondrial dynamics by SMAD. Molecular & Cellular Oncology. 2016;**3**(5):e1204492

[69] Kayhan M et al. Intrinsic TGF-beta signaling attenuates proximal tubule mitochondrial injury and inflammation in chronic kidney disease. Nature Communications. 2023;**14**(1):3236

[70] MacDonald BT, He X. Frizzled and LRP5/6 receptors for Wnt/beta-catenin signaling. Cold Spring Harbor Perspectives in Biology. 2012;**4**(12)

[71] MacDonald BT, Tamai K, He X. Wnt/beta-catenin signaling: Components, mechanisms, and diseases. Developmental Cell. 2009;**17**(1):9-26

[72] Anthony CC et al. Nuclear regulation of Wnt/beta-catenin Signaling: It's a complex situation. Genes (Basel). 2020;**11**(8)

[73] Kawakami T, Ren S, Duffield JS. Wnt signalling in kidney diseases: Dual roles

in renal injury and repair. The Journal of Pathology. 2013;**229**(2):221-231

[74] Wang Z et al. Beta-catenin promotes survival of renal epithelial cells by inhibiting Bax. Journal of the American Society of Nephrology. 2009;**20**(9):1919-1928

[75] Zhou D et al. Tubule-specific ablation of endogenous beta-catenin aggravates acute kidney injury in mice. Kidney International. 2012;**82**(5):537-547

[76] Clark PE et al. Beta-catenin and K-RAS synergize to form primitive renal epithelial tumors with features of epithelial Wilms' tumors. The American Journal of Pathology. 2011;**179**(6):3045-3055

[77] Akhmetshina A et al. Activation of canonical Wnt signalling is required for TGF-beta-mediated fibrosis. Nature Communications. 2012;**3**:735

[78] Caraci F et al. TGF-beta1 targets the GSK-3beta/beta-catenin pathway via ERK activation in the transition of human lung fibroblasts into myofibroblasts. Pharmacological Research. 2008;**57**(4):274-282

[79] Jian H et al. Smad3-dependent nuclear translocation of beta-catenin is required for TGF-beta1-induced proliferation of bone marrow-derived adult human mesenchymal stem cells. Genes & Development. 2006;**20**(6):666-674

[80] Liu YN et al. Regulatory mechanisms controlling human E-cadherin gene expression. Oncogene. 2005;**24**(56):8277-8290

[81] Sun BC et al. Expressions and significance of E-cadherin and beta-catenin in synovial sarcoma. Zhonghua Zhong Liu Za Zhi. 2005;**27**(12):727-730

[82] Choi SY et al. Class I HDACs specifically regulate E-cadherin expression in human renal epithelial cells. Journal of Cellular and Molecular Medicine. 2016;**20**(12):2289-2298

[83] Gottardi CJ, Wong E, Gumbiner BM. E-cadherin suppresses cellular transformation by inhibiting beta-catenin signaling in an adhesion-independent manner. The Journal of Cell Biology. 2001;**153**(5):1049-1060

[84] Westermann B. Bioenergetic role of mitochondrial fusion and fission. Biochimica et Biophysica Acta. 2012;**1817**(10):1833-1838

[85] Zhan M et al. Mitochondrial dynamics: Regulatory mechanisms and emerging role in renal pathophysiology. Kidney International. 2013;**83**(4):568-581

[86] Dudek J, Rehling P, van der Laan M. Mitochondrial protein import: Common principles and physiological networks. Biochimica et Biophysica Acta. 2013;**1833**(2):274-285

[87] Dukanovic J, Rapaport D. Multiple pathways in the integration of proteins into the mitochondrial outer membrane. Biochimica et Biophysica Acta. 2011;**1808**(3):971-980

[88] Jornayvaz FR, Shulman GI. Regulation of mitochondrial biogenesis. Essays in Biochemistry. 2010;**47**:69-84

[89] Kroemer G, Marino G, Levine B. Autophagy and the integrated stress response. Molecular Cell. 2010;**40**(2):280-293

[90] Granata S et al. Mitochondrial dysregulation and oxidative stress in patients with chronic kidney disease. BMC Genomics. 2009;**10**:388

[91] Mutsaers HA et al. Uremic toxins inhibit transport by breast cancer

resistance protein and multidrug resistance protein 4 at clinically relevant concentrations. PLoS One. 2011;**6**(4):e18438

[92] Chung KW et al. Mitochondrial damage and activation of the STING pathway Lead to renal inflammation and fibrosis. Cell Metabolism. 2019;**30**(4):784-799 e5

[93] Maekawa H et al. Mitochondrial damage causes inflammation via cGAS-STING Signaling in acute kidney injury. Cell Reports. 2019;**29**(5):1261-1273 e6

[94] Zuk A, Bonventre JV. Acute kidney injury. Annual Review of Medicine. 2016;**67**:293-307

[95] Silva-Garcia O, Valdez-Alarcon JJ, Baizabal-Aguirre VM. The Wnt/beta-catenin signaling pathway controls the inflammatory response in infections caused by pathogenic bacteria. Mediators of Inflammation. 2014;**2014**:310183

[96] Ma B, Hottiger MO. Crosstalk between Wnt/beta-catenin and NF-kappaB signaling pathway during inflammation. Frontiers in Immunology. 2016;**7**:378

[97] Duan Y et al. Beta-catenin activity negatively regulates bacteria-induced inflammation. Laboratory Investigation. 2007;**87**(6):613-624

[98] Canaud G, Bonventre JV. Cell cycle arrest and the evolution of chronic kidney disease from acute kidney injury. Nephrology, Dialysis, Transplantation. 2015;**30**(4):575-583

[99] Takahashi K et al. TGF-beta generates a population of cancer cells residing in G1 phase with high motility and metastatic potential via KRTAP2-3. Cell Reports. 2022;**40**(13):111411

[100] Wu DT et al. TGF-beta concentration specifies differential signaling profiles of growth arrest/differentiation and apoptosis in podocytes. Journal of the American Society of Nephrology. 2005;**16**(11):3211-3221

[101] Gewin L. The many talents of transforming growth factor-beta in the kidney. Current Opinion in Nephrology and Hypertension. 2019;**28**(3):203-210

[102] Liang J et al. The energy sensing LKB1-AMPK pathway regulates p27(kip1) phosphorylation mediating the decision to enter autophagy or apoptosis. Nature Cell Biology. 2007;**9**(2):218-224

[103] Ho KK, Myatt SS, Lam EW. Many forks in the path: Cycling with FoxO. Oncogene. 2008;**27**(16):2300-2311

[104] Thillainadesan G et al. TGF-beta-dependent active demethylation and expression of the p15ink4b tumor suppressor are impaired by the ZNF217/CoREST complex. Molecular Cell. 2012;**46**(5):636-649

[105] Feng XH, Lin X, Derynck R. Smad2, Smad3 and Smad4 cooperate with Sp1 to induce p15(Ink4B) transcription in response to TGF-beta. The EMBO Journal. 2000;**19**(19):5178-5193

[106] Heldin CH, Landstrom M, Moustakas A. Mechanism of TGF-beta signaling to growth arrest, apoptosis, and epithelial-mesenchymal transition. Current Opinion in Cell Biology. 2009;**21**(2):166-176

[107] Hannon GJ, Beach D. p15INK4B is a potential effector of TGF-beta-induced cell cycle arrest. Nature. 1994;**371**(6494):257-261

[108] Seoane J et al. TGFbeta influences Myc, Miz-1 and Smad to control the CDK

inhibitor p15INK4b. Nature Cell Biology. 2001;**3**(4):400-408

[109] Polyak K et al. Cloning of p27Kip1, a cyclin-dependent kinase inhibitor and a potential mediator of extracellular antimitogenic signals. Cell. 1994;**78**(1):59-66

[110] Seoane J et al. Integration of Smad and forkhead pathways in the control of neuroepithelial and glioblastoma cell proliferation. Cell. 2004;**117**(2):211-223

[111] Yang L et al. Epithelial cell cycle arrest in G2/M mediates kidney fibrosis after injury. Nature Medicine. 2010;**16**(5):535-543. 1p following 143

[112] DiRocco DP et al. CDK4/6 inhibition induces epithelial cell cycle arrest and ameliorates acute kidney injury. American Journal of Physiology. Renal Physiology. 2014;**306**(4):F379-F388

[113] Osaki Y et al. Blocking cell cycle progression through CDK4/6 protects against chronic kidney disease. JCI Insight. 2022;**7**(12)

[114] Medema RH et al. AFX-like Forkhead transcription factors mediate cell-cycle regulation by Ras and PKB through p27kip1. Nature. 2000;**404**(6779):782-787

[115] Gomis RR et al. A FoxO-Smad synexpression group in human keratinocytes. Proceedings of the National Academy of Sciences of the United States of America. 2006;**103**(34):12747-12752

[116] Li JM et al. Transforming growth factor beta activates the promoter of cyclin-dependent kinase inhibitor p15INK4B through an Sp1 consensus site. The Journal of Biological Chemistry. 1995;**270**(45):26750-26753

[117] Asada S et al. Mitogen-activated protein kinases, Erk and p38, phosphorylate and regulate Foxo1. Cellular Signalling. 2007;**19**(3):519-527

[118] Eijkelenboom A, Burgering BM. FOXOs: Signalling integrators for homeostasis maintenance. Nature Reviews. Molecular Cell Biology. 2013;**14**(2):83-97

[119] Lopez-Novoa JM et al. Common pathophysiological mechanisms of chronic kidney disease: Therapeutic perspectives. Pharmacology & Therapeutics. 2010;**128**(1):61-81

[120] Wuhl E, Schaefer F. Therapeutic strategies to slow chronic kidney disease progression. Pediatric Nephrology. 2008;**23**(5):705-716

[121] Patera F et al. Kidney fibrosis and oxidative stress: From molecular pathways to new pharmacological opportunities. Biomolecules. 2024;**14**(1)

[122] Zhao HJ et al. Effect of calcium channels blockers and inhibitors of the renin-angiotensin system on renal outcomes and mortality in patients suffering from chronic kidney disease: Systematic review and meta-analysis. Renal Failure. 2016;**38**(6):849-856

[123] Sugahara M, Tanaka T, Nangaku M. Prolyl hydroxylase domain inhibitors as a novel therapeutic approach against anemia in chronic kidney disease. Kidney International. 2017;**92**(2):306-312

[124] Shabaka A, Cases-Corona C, Fernandez-Juarez G. Therapeutic insights in chronic kidney disease progression. Frontiers in Medicine (Lausanne). 2021;**8**:645187

[125] Kansara A, Mubeen F, Shakil J. SGLT2 inhibitors in patients with chronic kidney disease and heart disease: A

literature review. Methodist DeBakey Cardiovascular Journal. 2022;**18**(4):62-72

[126] Border WA, Noble NA. Evidence that TGF-beta should be a therapeutic target in diabetic nephropathy. Kidney International. 1998;**54**(4):1390-1391

[127] Border WA, Noble NA. Interactions of transforming growth factor-beta and angiotensin II in renal fibrosis. Hypertension. 1998;**31**(1 Pt. 2):181-188

[128] Mallikarjuna P, Zhou Y, Landstrom M. The synergistic cooperation between TGF-beta and Hypoxia in cancer and fibrosis. Biomolecules. 2022;**12**(5)

[129] Zhao L, Zou Y, Liu F. Transforming growth factor-Beta1 in diabetic kidney disease. Frontiers in Cell and Development Biology. 2020;**8**:187

[130] Fuchs MAA et al. Inhibition of transforming growth factor beta1 signaling in resident interstitial cells attenuates profibrotic gene expression and preserves erythropoietin production during experimental kidney fibrosis in mice. Kidney International. 2021;**100**(1):122-137

Chapter 4

Chronic Kidney Disease of Unknown Origin in Sri Lanka: A Literature Review

Thushara Hewageegana, Nevil Rajakaruna and Chanaka Jayasinghe

Abstract

Sri Lanka is a tropical island situated south of India. A rise of incidence of chronic kidney disease (CKD) was reported from the dry zone of the country in the 1990s, which was not attributed to the traditional causes of CKD. It was named as chronic kidney disease of unknown origin (CKDu). We reviewed the literature to summarize the existing information on CKDu in Sri Lanka. The disease is more prevalent among farmers and has a unique locality. Numerous nephrotoxins, irrigation networks, genetic susceptibility, soil factor, and even bioterrorism as possible etiologies have been considered. Drinking water was proven to be hard and contain high fluoride levels, but toxins in food and water were controversial. Urine and tissues of affected patients contained some of the suspected toxins at higher levels. Though the majority of the researchers agreed on a toxic nephropathy, none of their hypotheses explain the clinical findings, and the unique locality of the disease, and its appearance in the 1990s. The absence of an identifiable cause has hampered controlling the disease. Careful use of agrochemicals and more researches to unravel the mystery is recommended.

Keywords: CKD, traditional causes of CKD, CKDu in Sri Lanka, dry zone, nephrotoxins, tubular- interstitial nephritis

1. Introduction

Chronic kidney disease is a global health problem which accounts for nearly 700 million active cases and 1.2 million deaths per year [1]. CKD is defined as abnormalities of kidney structure or function, present for >3 months, [2] with implications for health (**Table 1**).

The traditional causes for CKD include diabetes mellitus, glomerulonephritis, hypertension and structural abnormalities. However, chronic kidney diseases not attributed to any of the traditional etiologies have been reported throughout the world [3–5]. Because the cause of this disease is obscured, it is termed CKD of unknown etiology (CKDu). CKDu is well documented in areas including Central America [3], Eastern Europe [4], and Sri Lanka [5]. Many research papers have been published, and we linked those together to summarize the current knowledge on the

Either of the following present for > 3 months	
Markers of kidney damage (One or more)	• Urine albumin: creatinine ≥30 mg/g) • Urine sediment abnormalities • Electrolyte and other abnormalities due to tubular disorders • Abnormalities detected by histology • Structural abnormalities detected by imaging • History of kidney transplantation
Decreased Glomerular Filtration Rate (GFR)	<60 ml/min/1.73 m^2

Note that the table depicts the structural and functional abnormalities that account for CKD.

Table 1.
Criteria for CKD [2].

epidemiology, possible etiological factors, clinical and histopathological features of the disease. We obtained unpublished data from personal communications.

2. Sri Lanka and CKDu

Sri Lanka is a small island with a square area of 65,610 km^2 lying between latitudes 5° and 10° N, and longitudes 79° and 82° E, in the Indian Ocean, separated from the Indian subcontinent by the narrow marine strips, gulf of Mannar and the Palk Strait [6]. Sri Lanka has a tropical monsoon climate with three climatic zones; the wet zone, dry zone and the intermediate zone. The dry zone has an atmospheric temperature of 25–30°C with a mean annual rainfall <1500 mm (**Figure 1**) [8].

The majority of the Sri Lankan population depends on agriculture and related industries. Paddy (rice) is the main crop that is grown. A traditional and primitive form

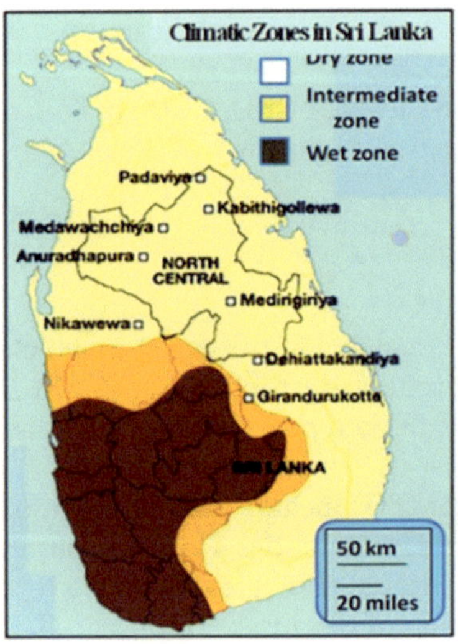

Figure 1.
A map of Sri Lanka illustrating the climatic zones of Sri Lanka: Dry, intermediate, and wet zones. Note that the dry zone is the largest zone on the island, involving nearly 2/3 of the territory [7].

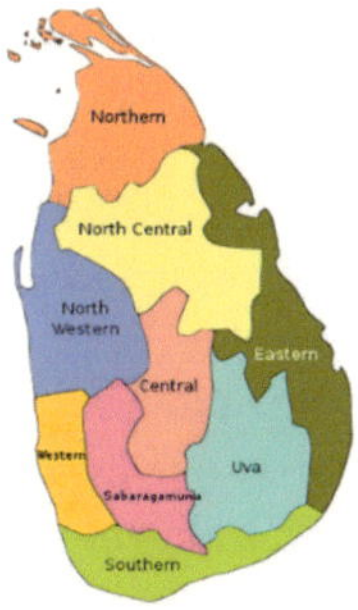

Figure 2.
Map of Sri Lanka illustrating its 9 provinces. Note that the NCP is extending in the dry zone.

of agriculture called 'Chena' cultivation where a farmer cultivates in a newly deforested land and moving on the next year to a fresh land is practiced in the country, mainly in the less populated dry zone. Agrochemicals including pesticides, herbicides and fertilizers are used all around the country [9]. Sri Lanka recorded the highest agrochemical consumption (287 units of agrochemicals per hectare) in the region [9].

Sri Lanka is divided into 9 administrative provinces and CKDu was first reported in the North-Central province (NCP) which is located in the dry zone of the country (see **Figure 2**).

The NCP is the largest province by area, with a population of 1,266,663, placing it the 3rd least populated province on the island. The NCP is the home to the ancient cities of Anuradhapura and Polonnaruwa, both of which were historical capitals of Sri Lanka for many centuries. From ancient days onwards, the area was famous for agriculture, mainly paddy. The insignia of the area is the vast number of medium and large-scale water tanks, some were built by ancient kings and some after the independence from the British rule in 1948. The area is supplied by irrigation water from 'Mahaweli', the longest river in the country, which was diverted in the 1970s.

Urinary tract disease was the 8th leading cause of in-hospital mortality in Sri Lanka in 2016 [10]. In contrast, it was the leading cause of hospital deaths in 2 districts that lie in the NCP of Sri Lanka, namely Anuradhapura and Polonnaruwa. The primary contributor to this relatively high death rate is the emergence of a new form of CKD-the CKDu, during the last few decades.

In Sri Lanka, CKDu was first reported in 1994 [11]. In 2009, the Sri Lankan ministry of health introduced criteria for case definition of CKDu. These included [12]:

1. No past history of, or current treatment for diabetes mellitus or chronic and/or severe hypertension, snake bites, urological disease or glomerulonephritis.

2. Normal glycosylated hemoglobin levels (< 6.5%).

3. Blood pressure < 160/100 mmHg untreated or < 140/90 mmHg on up to two antihypertensive agents.

3. Epidemiology of CKDu in Sri Lanka

CKDu was first reported in the NCP of the island [13] which is situated in the dry zone of the country. It was subsequently spread to the adjacent North-Western,

Eastern, and Uva provinces [12]. The endemic region covers approximately 24,000 km^2, providing shelter for about 3 million people. Out of that, about 2 million are at high risk of contracting CKDu (see **Figure 3**) [7].

The true prevalence is not known due to insufficient epidemiologic studies on the disease. A prevalence of 8–21% was reported in 2021 [11]. A point prevalence between 15.1 and 22.9% in 3 administrative districts including Anuradhapura and Polonnaruwa was reported in 2016 [14]. The World Health Organization (WHO) study in 2011 reported a prevalence of 15.6% in Anuradhapura, 20.6% in Medirigiriya in Polonnaruwa district and 22.9% in Giradurukotte in Badulla district [15]. The disease is prevalent in 11 out of 24 districts in Sri Lanka by 2017 [16]. About 400,000 CKDu cases were reported, with an estimated death toll of around 20,000 by 2013 [11].

There is a global male preponderance for CKDu [11]. A male preponderance for CKDu in Sri Lanka was reported in 2016 [14] which was confirmed by another study in 2017, with a prevalence of 17.5% in males and 7.6% in females [16]. However, an age-standardized prevalence of CKDu in Sri Lanka was at 12.9% in males and 16.9% in females, demonstrating a female preponderance [17]. The same cross-sectional study demonstrated a higher risk for the disease in females. In contrary, advanced CKDu was more frequent in Sri Lankan males. The prevalence CKDu stage 3 in males was 23.2% versus 7.4% in females; that of stage 4 was 22.0% versus 7.3% [17]. A more recent study in 2020 reporteor a male preponderance.

CKDu mostly affects the young and middle-aged in the world [5]. CKDu in Sri Lanka is more prevalent among the age group of 40–69 years [14]. CKDu principally affects communities in countries with developing economies [18]. Similarly, in Sri Lanka, lower socioeconomic groups are mainly affected [19].

Farming communities are the most affected stratum globally [19]. The Sri Lankan counterpart is also more common among the farmers indulge in 'Chena' and paddy cultivation [5]. Some researchers identified the primary victims of the epidemic as paddy farmers [1]. However, another study confirmed a higher risk for CKDu in 'Chena' cultivators than paddy farmers [17].

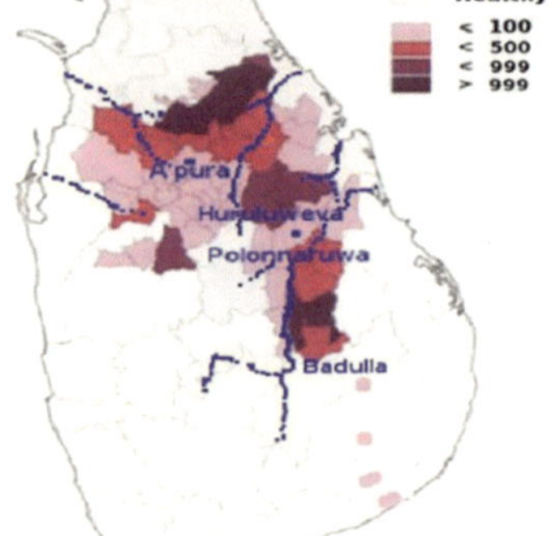

Figure 3.
Map of Sri Lanka depicting the distribution of CKDu [7]. Note that CKDu is entirely distributed in the dry zone and mainly involved the NCP. Note that one of the worst affected areas is situated outside the NCP in the adjacent North-Western province, and there are a few small pockets of CKDu in the southern parts of the island. The blue lines indicate rivers crossing the affected areas.

4. Clinical features

The CKDu is a disease that progresses slowly [20]. Patients are asymptomatic during most of the course of the disease [20]. Early detection of CKDu is a challenge [21]. Many victims of CKDu are not aware of being ill until the end stage [11].

Edema and hypertension occur late in the disease progression [14]. Hypertension was detected in half of the patients who underwent renal biopsies [22]. Anemia, immunodeficiency due to leucopenia and platelet dysfunctions are associated with the end stage CKDu like in any other end stage kidney disease [23].

Histopathology confirmed glomerular and tubulointerstitial disorder with vascular involvement [22]. Having examined 64 renal biopsies obtained from CKDu patients, researchers came to the following conclusions [22].

- Global sclerosis is the most common glomerular abnormality seen in renal biopsies.
- Glomerular enlargement was the second most common abnormality probably representing compensatory hypertrophy.
- Absence of endocapillary, extracapillary, or mesangial cell proliferation differentiates the lesion from chronic glomerulonephritis and diabetic glomerulosclerosis.
- PAS-positivity were not seen and immunocomplex disorders are less likely.
- Absence of tubulitis with invasion of tubular cells by inflammatory cells makes the etiology unlikely to be inflammation of tubular cells.
- Mononuclear infiltration is characteristic of the biopsies.
- Plasma cells and eosinophils that represent allergic nephritis were not observed.
- Interstitial fibrosis is common but tubular regeneration is uncommon.
- Out of vascular lesions, sclerosis, fibrous intimal thickening and arteriolar hyalinosis have been observed.

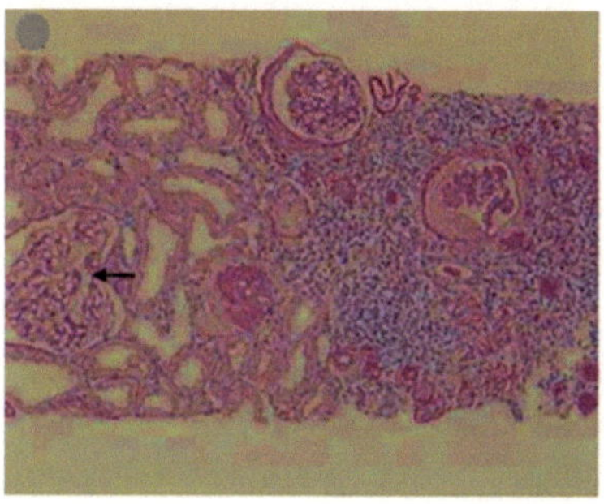

Figure 4.
Renal biopsy of a CKDu patient [22] showing interstitial inflammation, obsolescent glomeruli, tubular atrophy, and interstitial mononuclear cell infiltration on the right side. A hypertrophic nephron is seen on the left side (arrow) (PAS × 40).

- Histopathological features are compatible with tubular interstitial nephritis (see **Figure 4**).

The disease is characterized by tubular proteinuria, usually alpha-1 and beta-2 microglobulinuria, and high urine neutrophil gelatinase-associated lipocalin levels (>300 ng/mg creatinine) [12]. The available evidence on geographical and socioeconomic distribution of the disease hypothesizes that environmental, socioeconomic and occupational factors have a pivotal role to play as the main causative agents [12].

5. Etiology

Though the disease is believed to be a toxic nephropathy, conventional nephrotoxins such as lead, non-steroidal anti-inflammatory drugs, aminoglycosides, aristolochic acid and mycotoxins are highly unlikely as an isolated cause of CKDu in Sri Lanka [12]. A considerable number of researches have been conducted over the last couple of decades to identify an etiology of CKDu in Sri Lanka. However, no investigator has so far arrived at a solid conclusion on a definite causative factor of CKDu. A number of theories have been proposed which include pesticides, weedicides, chemical fertilizers, heavy metals, hard water, dehydration, fluoride, indigenous medications, illicit alcohol, beetle chewing, irrigation work, algae, fungal toxins, bioterrorism and pets [1, 5, 24]. Though majority of the researchers agreed on a toxic nephropathy, none of their hypothesis so far could explain the clinical, biochemical, histopathological findings, and the unique geographical distribution of the disease and its appearance in the mid-1990s.

6. Agrochemicals

Green revolution in the 1960s completely revolutionized the agricultural system in Sri Lanka with replacement of the traditional eco-friendly farming with modernized machinery, technology, hybrid seeds and agrochemicals. Change of economic policies in 1977 in Sri Lanka allowed to importation and application of agrochemicals on a large scale [12]. Agrochemicals are imported to Sri Lanka as finished products, or as materials which are formulated locally [15].

Estimated pesticide use in Sri Lanka is around 0.308 kg and around 1.056 kg per hectare of arable lands and actively cultivated lands, respectively. Due to the influence of local traders and availability of pesticides in a large number of trade names, farmers inadvertently overuse the same active ingredient from different products. In 2010, WHO recommended taking immediate steps to limit agrochemical use [9].

Further, Sri Lankan farmers do not consistently utilize personal protective equipment like face masks, gloves and body aprons while engaged in application of poisonous agrochemicals. However, occupational pesticide exposure was not found to be significant risk factors for CKDu in Sri Lanka [5]. Further, Sri Lanka uses only about 1/5 to 1/10 the agrochemicals per hectare used by New Zealand (1836 kg/hectare in 2013) which is free of chronic kidney disease of unknown etiology [25].

Organophosphates are the commonest pesticide used in Sri Lanka (see **Table 2**). The earliest CKDu study in Sri Lanka evaluating pesticide exposure revealed a significant difference in red cell acetylcholinesterase levels: exposed CKD

Name of the chemical	Use	kg or L approved for import
Glyphosate (acid equivalent)	Herbicide	5,295,082
Propanil	Herbicide	995,310
MCPA	Herbicide	686,375
Mancozeb	Fungicide	671,504
Chlorpyrifos	Pesticide	420,008
Carbofuran	Pesticide	299,000
Diazinon	Pesticide	196,735
Profenofos	Pesticide	140,768
Carbosulfan	Pesticide	107,000
Pretilachlor + Pyribenzoxim	Herbicide	102,297

The table indicates that the commonest herbicide imported is glyphosate (acid equivalent) while the commonest imported pesticide and fungicide are chlorpyrifos and mancozeb respectively.

Table 2.
Leading pesticides, herbicides and fungicides imported to Sri Lanka in 2012.

(18.6 U/g) < unexposed CKD (26) < exposed non-CKD (29.1) < non-exposed non-CKD (32.6) and the authors suggested further investigations to assess the possible association between pesticide use and CKDu [26].

Pesticide residues were detected in the urine of CKDu patients. The frequency of detection of 2,4-D, 3,5,6-trichloropyridinol (metabolite of chlorpyrifos), p-nitrophenol (metabolite of parathion), 1-naphthol (metabolite of carbaryl naphthalene), 2-naphthol (metabolite of naphthalene), glyphosate, AMPA (metabolite of glyphosate) was 33%, 70%, 58%, 100%, 100%, 65% and 28% respectively. p-nitrophenol excretors did not have CKD while 10.5% each of 1-naphthol and 2-naphthol excretors had CKD [17].

Glyphosate is the most widely used weedicide in Sri Lanka (see **Table 2**). Glyphosate was thought to be readily degradable to non-toxic compounds and has a typical half-life of 47 days [12, 27]. However been extremely water-soluble, glyphosate readily escapes into the environment causing contamination of groundwater and accumulation in the plant tissues impeding its elimination [28]. It has descaling properties and bind to metals like calcium and magnesium [12]. Glyphosate metal complex increases the half-life of the herbicide in the soil up to 7 years or even up to 22 years [12]. The soil and groundwater in the CKDu affected area are rich in calcium and magnesium and have the capacity to retain glyphosate in them for a long period. Though there are no human studies on glyphosate nephrotoxicity, animal trials have shown to cause nephrotoxicity in mice [29]. Further, glyphosate can explain the unique geographical distribution of CKDu in areas with hard water and occurrence of the epidemic in the 1990s [12].

However, some researchers point out that there is no evidence to confirm that glyphosate has any adverse effect on kidneys with the amounts that are recommended for farming activities. Further, glyphosate binds soil particles and form insoluble complexes with calcium and magnesium [25] making the possibility of leaching into water resources and getting absorbed from the human intestine very remote. Glyphosate make no complexes with cadmium and arsenic and has no role of been a vehicle for those cations [25].

7. Hard water

Crystal-tubular nephropathy (CTN) has been inadvertently categorized under the umbrella of CKDu [18]. CTN is due to natural geogenic water contamination. Consumption of hard water obtained from deep-dug wells and tube wells over decades is required for its manifestations. The CTN prevailing area are identified north of the equator close to it [18] and Sri Lanka is situated in that geographic locality. Scanty rainfall and hot climate further concentrate the minerals in the groundwater by evaporation. Hard water is unpalatable and as a result, peasants consume lesser amounts of water subjecting themselves to chronic dehydration, which favors calcium phosphate crystal formation in renal parenchyma [18]. Histological and preliminary electron microscopic findings confirmed the deposition of calcium phosphate in kidney tissue [18].

Hardness of water in endemic areas is mainly due calcium, magnesium, strontium and iron [12]. Ninety six percent of the CKDu patients had consumed hard water obtained from ground wells for at least five years [12]. Places with high ground water hardness and the geographical distribution of the CKDu in Sri Lanka are well correlated [12].

People who consume natural springs located in the CKDu endemic area and those who consume treated water and centrally purified pipe borne water are less affected by the disease [12]. However, northern province with the maximum hardness of water in the entire island has a low prevalence of the disease [12]. **Figure 5** illustrates the distribution of hardness of water in Sri Lanka.

8. Fluoride (F)

Hard water in areas where CKDu is known to contain higher levels of fluoride [7]. The presence of fluoride stabilizes calcium phosphate nano-minerals and permit their

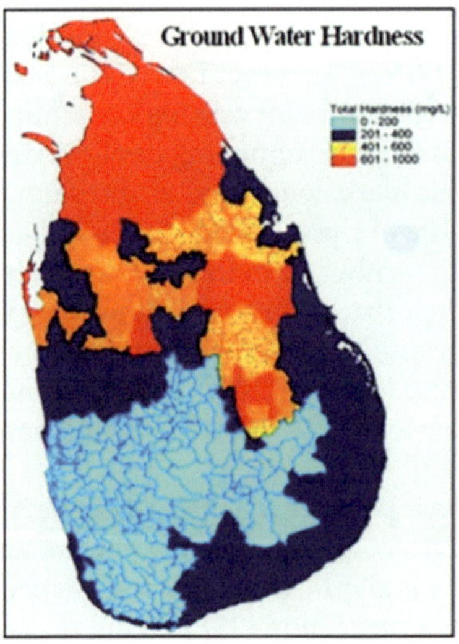

Figure 5.
*Map of Sri Lanka illustrating the hardness of water. Note that the hardness is tallying with the CKDu prevalence (see **Figure 3**) except in the Northern province [7].*

Area	Number of samples	Average F	Maximum F
Giradurukotte	38	0.74	2.14
Nikawewa- Siyabalangamuwa	45	1.41	5.30
Medawachchiya	22	1.02	4.9
Padaviya-Sri Pura	14	0.50	1.96
Vavuniya	08	0.63	1.18
Huruluwewa	14	1.03	1.68

Note that Nikawewa- Siyabalangamuwa having the highest level though situated outside the most affected NCP.

Table 3.
Fluoride content of ground water in some affected area in mg/L [31].

growth in the renal parenchyma [18]. The ground water fluoride levels and the CKDu distribution has a close relationship [30].

In the mid-1980s, the rise of the water table in the affected area resulted from diversion of water from new irrigation project [30]. This led to leaching of more fluorides to ground water from fluoride rich minerals in the earth [30].

Fluoride levels in ground water in the affected areas in Sri Lanka exceed the World Health Organization (WHO) recommended limit of 0.5 mg/L for tropical countries (see **Table 3**).

The incidence of dental fluorosis is common even in areas with fluoride levels below the statuary upper limit [31]. This raises the suspicion of other sources of fluoride toxicity. Black tea is rich in fluoride and is a popular beverage among farming communities [31]. High content of fluoride in groundwater results in higher fluoride contents in local food crops subjecting the consumers to higher fluoride intake [30]. Presence of calcium and magnesium ions which is typical of the region enhances the nephrotoxicity of fluoride [1, 25]. Further, cations like cadmium which is presumed to contaminate drinking water in the endemic areas also aggravates fluoride induced renal failure [1].

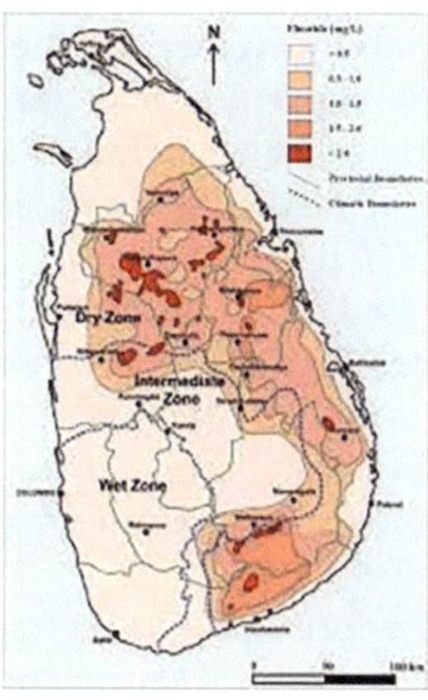

Figure 6.
*Map of Sri Lanka showing the concentration of fluoride in ground water. Note that fluoride concentrations closely agree with CKDu prevalence shown in **Figure 3** [33].*

However, serum fluoride concentrations of most of the healthy and stages 1 and 2 CKDu patients were below the upper cut-off value of 50 µg/L [32]. Late stages of CKDu patients had serum fluoride above the normal range [32]. This is explained by decreased fluoride excretion in advanced CKD and further deteriorating the kidney functions [32]. This indicates that increased serum fluoride levels in CKDu patients is the effect rather than the cause of CKDu (**Figure 6**).

9. Chronic dehydration

Inhabitants of tropical countries who indulge in manual outdoor activities expose themselves to high atmospheric temperature and develop chronic dehydration. Chronic occupational heat stress and dehydration are now thought to be the key etiologic factors for CKDu [27]. Chronic dehydration is a promoting factor for the development of crystal nephropathy [18]. In Central America the main focus of attention for researches in CKDu is dehydration and heat stress, but it has been paid less attention in Asia [11] including Sri Lanka.

The possible pathophysiological mechanism of CKD in chronic dehydration includes sub-clinical rhabdomyolysis, hyperuricemia and hyperuricosuria, hyperosmolarity and vasopressin effects [11]. Hard water in the CKDu prevailing area makes the water unpalatable [18] and as a result people drink less which causes dehydration in a vicious cycle.

The dehydration hypothesis, however, cannot fully elucidate the low disease prevalence in the neighboring Northern province of Sri Lanka, where the conditions are warmer and drier than the endemic areas [34].

10. Heavy metals

10.1 Aluminum

With its known nephrotoxic effect aluminum [5] is implicated as a possible cause for CKDu. Substandard aluminum cooking utensils and containers used to store drinking water are a possible source of aluminum toxicity. Boiling of water in those containers which is done to kill pathogens increase the risk of aluminum leach and contamination of water [5]. Triple superphosphate fertilizers contain aluminum as impurities which is another source of water pollution with aluminum [34]. Aluminum concentration of drinking water in the disease prevalent areas was above the statuary upper limit of the WHO which is 10 µg/L [34].

Aluminum leaching is increased when fluoride concentration is more than 1 mg/L [35] which is encountered with the ground water of the endemic areas (see **Table 3**). Leaching of aluminum is increased under acidic conditions regardless of the fluoride content of water [24]. Inhabitants of the endemic areas use an extract of an acidic fruit *Tamarindus indica* that contain organic acids to clean aluminum containers.

However, according to some reports, aluminum fluoride complex is not likely to be more toxic than fluoride itself [25]. Further, serum and urine studies do not suggest aluminum as a causative agent for CKDu [15].

10.2 Cadmium

Cadmium is a heavy metal with well-known nephrotoxic properties. Several studies reported considerable amounts of cadmium in the biological samples of CKDu patients [1]. A significant level of cadmium was found in rice, vegetables and raw tobacco sold in CKDu endemic areas [12]. The same study revealed that triple phosphate fertilizers imported to Sri Lanka are contaminated with significant amounts of cadmium [12].

Cadmium could enter the body through drinking water, food and tobacco [34]. Researchers demonstrated a cadmium level of 0.03 to 0.06 mg/L in reservoir water which is well above the statuary upper limit of 0.005 mg/L recommended by the US Environment Protection Agency [19]. Lotus (*Nelumbo nucifera*) root which is consumed by the local people contained cadmium at 253.82 mg/kg [36]. The provisional tolerable weekly intake of cadmium, based on the extreme exposure for rice and fish, was also found to be high in the region [36].

Urinary excretion of cadmium is a consistent marker of chronic exposure to cadmium [34]. The mean concentration of cadmium in urine in CKDu patients was significantly higher (1.039 mg/g) compared to controls in the endemic (0.646 mg/g) and non-endemic areas. (0.345 mg/g) [34].

Presence of cadmium and fluorides both mutually enhanced their toxicities by three times in soft water [34]. A significantly higher cadmium concentration was also seen in the nails of CKDu patients [17].

However, cadmium levels in drinking water of CKDu patients in the NCP was found to lie below WHO recommended statuary upper limit of 5 μg/L [34]. Also, the dietary load of cadmium was similar in the endemic areas, and in the non-endemic areas which does not explain the unique distribution of CKDu. The cadmium levels found in the rice grown in the rain fed wet zone exceed the amounts in the dry zone by 40–60% [25]. He also pointed out that even an extremely contaminated sample of fertilizers containing 50 mg of cadmium per kg will take 1.2 millennia for the soil to impregnate with cadmium to a hazardous level [25].

10.3 Arsenic

Arsenic is not a well-known nephrotoxic agent. However, some researchers found that it is potentially nephrotoxic in the presence of calcium and magnesium ions [12]. which are typical of the ground water in the endemic areas. They confirmed the presence of arsenic in toxic concentrations in nails hair and urine of CKDu patients and healthy individuals living in the affected areas. They proposed that the origin of arsenic is poor quality agrochemicals rather than geological as is seen in some countries like Bangladesh [12]. The WHO found approximately 88% of CKDu patients had urine arsenic >21 μg/g creatinine, which is above the nephrotoxic limit [37]. Most crops do not take up much arsenic from the ground, except rice which is the main staple in the country [7]. However, arsenic levels in the rice samples from both CKDu endemic and non-endemic areas were well below the statuary upper limit for Codex standard [38].

Further, no arsenic was found in reservoir water in the endemic region [36] while Gibbs free energy calculations confirmed that arsenic in the presence of fluoride and hardness which is typical of the area, has no synergistic effect, in fact, may expect to be less nephrotoxic [25].

11. Other heavy metals

Possibility of lead, chromium, nickel, cobalt, copper, vanadium and strontium toxicity as a causative factor of CKDu has been investigated [36]. Lead levels in urine samples and tissue biopsies of patients were above the expected amounts [25].

Glyphosate makes complexes with nickel cobalt, lead and vanadium [12]. This complex enters the body in water, food or by inhalation to cause nephrotoxicity. Rice and soil in the paddy lands in the CKDu endemic area are rich in chromium, iron, nickel and cobalt. Further, triple phosphate fertilizers available in Sri Lanka found contaminated with significant amounts of heavy metals [12].

However, other researchers contradicted above findings. They found a negligible amount of heavy metals found in the water and soil in the affected areas [17, 25]. Urine concentrations of copper, zinc, and titanium in CKDu cases were within normal limits [17]. Further, there was no significant difference in urine lead concentrations in CKDu cases compared to controls [17]. Serum chromium and strontium levels were within normal limits [17].

11.1 Selenium

Selenium is thought to have a nephroprotective effect at a concentration of 90 μg/L. and about two-thirds of CKDu subjects had selenium levels below this cut-off value [17].

12. Blue-green algae (Cyanobacteria)

The NCP is studded with an interconnecting irrigation system where the farming lands are watered by canals from reservoirs. The reservoirs are filled by the Mahaweli river which is fed mainly from the central hill country which is free from CKDu. However, agrochemicals washouts are likely to get accumulated in the low-lying reservoirs.

Algae infestation in the reservoirs could have been the result of fertilizer washouts, global warming and diversion of river water which alters the local fauna and flora. Algae growing in open water in the region were suspected as a cause for CKDu.

Blue-green algae synthesize cyanotoxins including microcystin, cylindrospermopsin and deoxy-cylindrospermopsin, all of which are acute nephrotoxins [34].

However, the affected community does not obtain drinking water from irrigation canals or reservoirs [34]. Further, Padaviya reservoir providing water to one of the most affected CKDu areas has shown low levels of cyanotoxins [34]. Also, ground water in shallow wells and tube wells in the CKDu endemic area is free from cyanotoxins [34].

13. Mycotoxins

Mycotoxins are linked to CKDu in some settings. These toxins include aflatoxins ochratoxins and fumonisins [39]. They enter the human body through contaminated cereals, beans, spices, dried fruits, nuts and oilseeds. All three toxins were detected in CKDu patients in Sri Lanka with relatively higher levels than normal counterparts living in the same area [40]. Most patients were detected with ochratoxins [40].

However, levels in dietary mycotoxin levels were found in insignificant levels in CKDu endemic areas [14]. The evidence for mycotoxins as a causative agent for CKDu in Sri Lanka is inadequate up to date [14].

14. Irrigation networks

Some researchers have suggested an association between the CKDu and irrigation network in the area, particularly the diverted water from the Mahaweli river [7]. Mahaweli, the longest river in the island was planned to divert to the dry zone in 1960s and the process was accelerated in 1977.

The Mahaweli project is the one that irrigates areas with the largest number of CKDu patients (**Figure 7**) [7].

The water diverted from the Mahaweli river is polluted with large quantities of washed-off agrochemicals and other materials coming from the hill country [7]. Also, the Mahaweli project led to inadvertent exposure of heavy metals deposited in the deeper layers of soil and other potential contaminants, which were returned to the surface water systems [7].

15. Bioterrorism

Sri Lanka was in a mid of a civil for from 1983 up to 2019. Several separatist armed groups fought with Sri Lankan state military forces to make an independent state for Sri Lankan Tamils claiming certain administrative districts of the island. The prevalence of CKDu is low in admirative districts claimed by the separatists. This raised the suspicion of bioterrorism. However, as the Sri Lankan armed forces realized that separatist groups make explosives using agrochemicals, they were banned to the war zone. This led to the use of a comparatively low number of agrochemicals particularly in the northern part of Sri Lanka. This is the most likely reason why CKDu is not extended to the war zone of the yester era (**Figure 8**) [12].

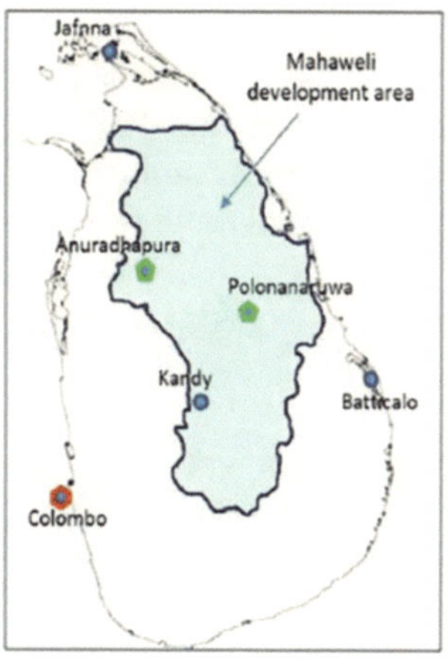

Figure 7.
*Map of Sri Lanka demonstrating Mahaweli fed areas. Note that the CKDu prevalence (see **Figure 3**) is closely related to the Mahaweli feeding areas [7].*

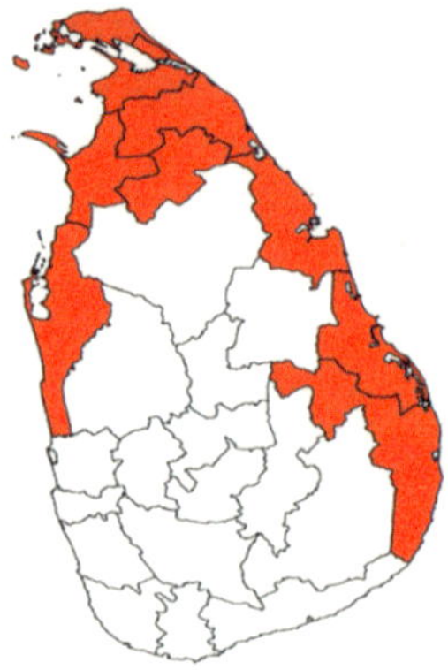

Figure 8.
The shaded area in red indicates the territory claimed by the separatists. Note that the disease has not spread (see ***Figure 3****) into that territory [41].*

16. Alcohol, tobacco and betel

Consumption of alcohol and tobacco and betel chewing is practiced among Sri Lankans. Betel leaves are chewed with other condiments like arecanut tobacco and lime.

Regular alcohol intake aggravates chronic dehydration which is implicated in CKDu [18]. Exposure to nephrotoxic heavy metals through alcohol is possible [1]. However, alcohol consumption was not found to be a significant risk factor for CKDu [5].

Tobacco as a possible source of heavy metal poisoning implicated in CKDu was proposed [1] and a statistically significant association with CKDu was observed with chewing betel [5].

17. Herbal medications

Balkan nephropathy was renamed aristolochic acid nephropathy having *Aristolochia clematitis*, a plant that contaminates wheat, been confirmed as the cause [12]. *Aristolochia indica* (Sapsanda/Sassanda in local language Sinhalese) is a plant belongs to the same botanical family is found in Sri Lanka (see **Figure 9**). This plant is used in indigenous and traditional medicine. WHO reported 60 indigenous medical prescriptions in Sri Lanka containing Aristolochia [37]. A personal conversation with Sisika Jagoda-Arachchi -a traditional medical practitioner from Thalawa,

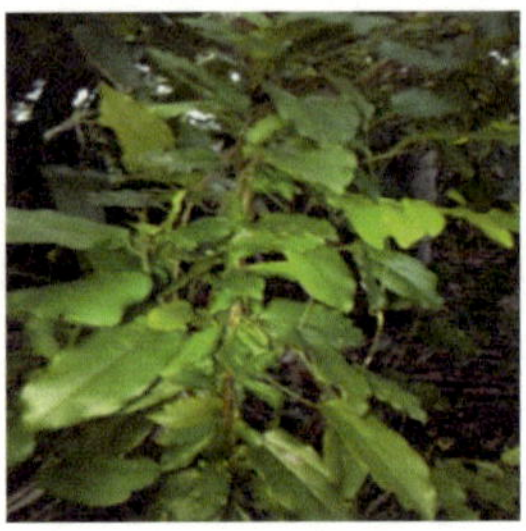

Figure 9.
Aristolochia indica plant growing wild in the NCP of Sri Lanka.

Anuradhapura (January 2024) revealed that the extracts of this plant are used as oral medications to treat snake envenomation and worm infestation.

However, urothelial cancers that are associated with aristolochic acid nephropathy is not seen in the Sri Lankan counterpart [12]. Therefore herbal medications and aristolochic acid contaminated foods is an irrational suspect for CKDu in Sri Lanka [12].

18. Genetic susceptibility

Clustering of disease, as happens in CKDu, suggests an unexpected influence from either genetics, environment, or both. These hotspots likely signify the locations where genetic susceptibility and environmental triggers share the most overlap [41]. A genome-wide association study was conducted to determine the genetic contributors, and genetic susceptibility was identified as a major risk factor for CKDu in Sri Lanka [42, 43]. Presence of numerous rare variants contributing CKDu is also likely [43].

19. Soil factor

Sri Lanka has seven main soil groups, and red brown soil is the type found in the dry zone (**Figure 10**) [44].

20. Screening program

In 2014, a committee for the control of CKDu was appointed by the state to plan a systematic screening program for early diagnosis [45]. Epidemiology Unit of the Ministry of Health Sri Lanka, selected fifty sentinel hospitals based on disease burden, media reports, and public concerns [45]. Based on hospital data, the NCP and

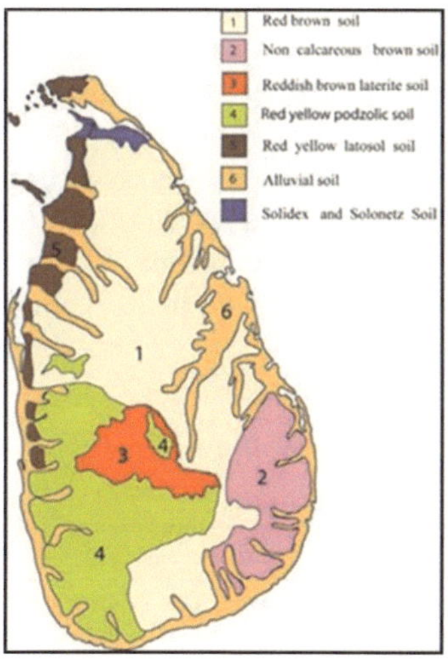

Figure 10.
*Map of Sri Lanka illustrating the distribution of soil. Note that the endemic areas of CKDu (see **Figure 3**) are mainly located in regions with red brown soil [44].*

several adjacent areas were identified as high-risk areas and some referral hospitals were selected [45].

The primary target group in endemic areas includes those who are above the age of twenty years and in non-endemic areas, those who are above the age of thirty [45]. Those who are suffering from acute illness, pregnant women and women during menstruation are considered as exclusion criteria for screening [45].

The aims of the screening program include detection of asymptomatic individuals in the early stages of the chronic kidney disease, assessing the disease burden of CKD/CKDu in the entire country giving priority to CKDu endemic areas, referring the positive cases for specialized centers and identifying factors associated with CKDu [45].

Field screening centers testing for serum creatinine with an estimated glomerular filtration rate (eGFR) calculated by CKD-EPI formula, measuring urine albumin creatinine ratio (UACR) on an early morning urine sample and measuring blood pressure have been established [45]. A blood pressure above 140 mmHg and 90 mmHg and/or serum creatinine above the age specific reference ranges and/or eGFR below 60 ml/1.73 m^2/min, UACR 30 mg/g of creatinine is taken as positive for screening for CKD and will be referred to a specialized unit for further evaluation [45].

21. Treatment

CKDu in Sri Lanka is managed as any other CKD. Dialysis and transplant are offered to end stage CKDu patients. Dialysis units are in operation at Teaching Hospital Anuradhapura (THA) and District General Hospital Polonnaruwa, while dialysis centers available at in Nort- Central province include Padaviya, Kebithigollewa Medawachchiya, Thambuththegama, Medirigiriya and Hingurangoda [46].

22. Current situation

Sri Lanka continues to diagnose new cases of CKDu in the new decade and the apparent reduction in the number of new cases in 2020 and 2021 in comparison to 2018 is probably due to decreased number of screenings in the mid of the Covid-19 epidemic (see **Table 4**).

Data has not been updated after 2021. We obtained unpublished data from Dr. PLGH Liyanage- medical officer, renal care unit, provincial directorate health services, NCP in January 2024 in a personal communication. In 2022, 2781 cases were positive out of 33,510 who were screened and in 2023 3868 were positive out of 64,026.

Year	Anuradhapura	Polonnaruwa
2018	2377	1048
2019	867	1165
2020	337	631
2021	1360	682

Table 4.
Newly diagnosed CKD patients in the NCP [46].

Year	Anuradhapura	Polonnaruwa
2018	No data available	253
2019	276	276
2020	659	255
2021	660	376

Table 5.
Number of CKD deaths in two districts in the NCP [46].

Year	Anuradhapura excluding THA	Polonnaruwa
2016	63	126
2017	81	160
2018	132	196
2019	165	279
2020	191	311
2021	266	354

Table 6.
Number of dialysis patients in two districts of the NCP [46].

Number of deaths from CKDu continue to rise in the NCP as depicted in **Table 5**.

The number of patients undergoing dialysis is also on the rise in the NCP (see **Table 6**).

However, these data reveal only the tip of the iceberg as some CKDu patients have the access to the dialysis units other than those placed in the NCP and the data has not included the number of dialysis performed at Teaching Hospital Anuradhapura.

23. Discussion

A definite cause of CKDu in Sri Lanka is yet to recognize. But most probably it is multifactorial in origin and therefore the term 'CKD of multi-factorial origin' (CKD-mfo) has been proposed. 32] CKDu has emerged as a dreaded disease affecting the farming communities of Sri Lanka who are the backbone of the national economy. The prevalence of CKDu is on the rise and the disease has a major negative impact on the economy of the country which is based mainly on agriculture.

Researchers confirmed contamination of water and food with potential nephrotoxins which entails long lasting disastrous consequences on health. Human interventions in farming industry constantly disrupt the nature leads to ecological imbalances with an exposure of toxic elements and emergence of new diseases like CKDu.

Traditional agriculture was used for generations on the island. Organic agriculture which is echo friendly has been proposed by various researchers [32] was inadvertently introduced to the country in 2020 ending up in a failure [47].

Most researches done were based on narrow or single cause hypotheses, ignoring potential interactions and synergistic effects of various agents. Though no potential single etiology for CKDu was identified, those suspected agents may be associated with the disease and may have an additive or synergistic pathological effect to cause CKDu. This is likely even when the toxin levels are well below the upper statuary limits.

Because CKDu is likely to be caused by adverse alterations in the environment including soil, water and food, there is no medical solution to eliminate it. Instead, health education and safe agrochemical handing are indicated in preventing CKDu.

24. Conclusions

The current epidemic of CKDu is most probably multifactorial in origin and environmentally acquired. Provision of purified drinking water, health education and proper handling of agrochemicals is important.

After three decades of researches in CKDu, Sri Lanka still need extensive epidemiological study to identify the root cause, disease burden and spread of CKDu.

Acknowledgements

We thank HPP Kumari (Tract 4, Near the bus stand, Rajangana, Sri Lanka) for locating an *Aristolochia indica* plant.

Conflict of interest

The authors declare no conflict of interest.

Author details

Thushara Hewageegana*, Nevil Rajakaruna and Chanaka Jayasinghe
Department of Chemical Pathology, Teaching Hospital Anuradhapura, Sri Lanka

*Address all correspondence to: hewageegana@gmail.com

References

[1] Imbulana S, Oguma K. Groundwater as a potential cause of chronic kidney disease of unknown etiology (CKDu) in Sri Lanka: A review. Journal of Water and Health. 2021;**19**(3):393-410. DOI: 10.2166/wh.2021.079

[2] Levin A, Stevens PE. Summary of KDIGO 2012 CKD Guideline: behind the scenes, need for guidance, and a framework for moving forward. Kidney International. 2014;**85**(1):49-61. DOI: 10.1038/ki.2013.444

[3] Correa-Rotter R, Wesseling C, Johnson RJ. CKD of unknown origin in Central America: The case for a Mesoamerican nephropathy. American Journal of Kidney Diseases. 2014;**63**(3):506-520. DOI: 10.1053/j.ajkd.2013.10.062

[4] Pavlović NM. Balkan endemic nephropathy-current status and future perspectives. Clinical Kidney Journal. 2013;**6**(3):257-265. DOI: 10.1093/ckj/sft049

[5] Pry M, Jackson W, Rupasinghe R, et al. A pilot case-control study using a one health approach to evaluate behavioral, environmental, and occupational risk factors for chronic kidney disease of unknown etiology in Sri Lanka. One Health Outlook. 2021;**3**:4. DOI: 10.1186/s42522-020-00034-3

[6] Wikipedia, the free encyclopedia. Sri Lanka [cited December 13, 2023]. 2023. Available from: https://en.wikipedia.org/wiki/Sri_Lanka

[7] Wimalawansa SJ. Escalating chronic kidney diseases of multi-factorial origin (CKD-mfo) in Sri Lanka: Causes, solutions, and recommendations-update and responses. Environmental Health and Preventive Medicine. 2015;**20**:152-157. DOI: 10.1007/s12199-015-0447-5

[8] Department of Meteorology Sri Lanka. Climate in Sri Lanka. 2000. Available from: http://www.meteo.gov.lk/index.php?option=com_content&view=article&id=94&Itemid=310&lang=en#4-northeast-monsoon-season-december-february [Accessed: June 6, 2020]

[9] Sri Lanka. Highest Agrochemical User-Government Medical Officers Association. 2013. Available from: https://www.gmoa.lk/sri-lanka-highest-agrochemical-user/

[10] Wijewickrama ES, Gunawardena N, Jayasinghe S, Herath C. CKD of unknown Etiology (CKDu) in Sri Lanka: A multilevel clinical case definition for surveillance and epidemiological studies. Kidney International Report. 2019;**4**(6):781-785. DOI: 10.1016/j.ekir.2019.03.020

[11] Paidi G, Iroshani Jayarathna AI, Salibindla DBAMR, Amirthalingam J, Karpinska-Leydier K, Alshowaikh K, et al. Chronic kidney disease of unknown origin: A mysterious epidemic. Cureus. 2021;**13**(8):e17132. DOI: 10.7759/cureus.17132

[12] Jayasumana C, Gunatilake S, Senanayake P. Glyphosate, hard water and nephrotoxic metals: Are they the culprits behind the epidemic of chronic kidney disease of unknown etiology in Sri Lanka? International Journal of Environmental Research and Public Health. 2014;**11**(2):2125-2147. DOI: 10.3390/ijerph110202125

[13] Ranasinghe AV, Kumara GWGP, Karunarathna RH, et al. The incidence,

prevalence and trends of chronic kidney disease and chronic kidney disease of uncertain aetiology (CKDu) in the north central province of Sri Lanka: An analysis of 30,566 patients. BMC Nephrology. 2019;**20**:338. DOI: 10.1186/s12882-019-1501-0

[14] Rajapakse S, Shivanthan MC, Selvarajah M. Chronic kidney disease of unknown etiology in Sri Lanka. International Journal of Occupational Environmental Health. 2016;**22**(3):259-264. DOI: 10.1080/10773525.2016.1203097

[15] Wanigasuriya K. Chronic kidney disease of unknown aetiology in Sri Lanka; a journey to unravel the mystery. Journal of the Ceylon College of Physicians. 2020;**51**:76-81

[16] Epidemiology Unit of Ministry of Health, Nutrition and Indigenous Medicine. World Health Organization. National Science Foundation of Sri Lanka. Prevalence and risk factors for CKDu in the district of Anuradhapura. 2017

[17] Jayatilake N, Mendis S, Maheepala P, et al. Chronic kidney disease of uncertain aetiology: Prevalence and causative factors in a developing country. BMC Nephrology. 2013;**14**:180. DOI: 10.1186/1471-2369-14-180

[18] Wimalawansa SJ, Dissanayake CB. Nanocrystal-induced chronic tubular-nephropathy in tropical countries: Diagnosis, mitigation, and eradication. European Journal of Medical Research. 2023;**28**:221. DOI: 10.1186/s40001-023-01162-yut B

[19] Wanigasuriya KP, Peiris-John RJ, Wickremasinghe R. Chronic kidney disease of unknown aetiology in Sri Lanka: Is cadmium a likely cause? BMC Nephrology. 2011;**12**:32. DOI: 10.1186/1471-2369-12-32

[20] Jayasumana MA, Paranagama PA, Dahanayake KS, Wijewardena KC, Amarasinghe MD, Fonseka SI. Possible link of chronic arsenic toxicity to chronic kidney disease of unknown etiology in Sri Lanka. JNSR. 2013;**3**:64-73

[21] Selvarajah M, Weeratunga P, Sivayoganthan S, Rathnatunga N, Rajapakse S. Clinicopathological correlates of chronic kidney disease of unknown etiology in Sri Lanka. Indian Journal of Nephrology. 2016;**26**(5):357-363. DOI: 10.4103/0971-4065.167280

[22] Nanayakkara S, Senevirathna ST, Abeysekera T, Chandrajith R, Ratnatunga N, Gunarathne ED, et al. An integrative study of the genetic, social and environmental determinants of chronic kidney disease characterized by tubulointerstitial damages in the north central region of Sri Lanka. Journal of Occupational Health. 2014;**56**(1):28-38. DOI: 10.1539/joh.13-0172-oa

[23] Gunawickrama SHNP, Hewavitharana KIG, Nanayakkara PGCL, Gunawickrama KBS. Chronic kidney disease of unknown Etiology (CKDu) in Sri Lanka: Hematological changes and pro-inflammation suggest likely predictors of advance disease, as renal outcomes show prevalent normoalbuminuria. Diseases. 2021;**10**(1):2. DOI: 10.3390/diseases10010002

[24] Ileperuma OA, Dharmagunawardhane HA, Herath KPRP. Dissolution of aluminium from sub-standard utensils under high fluoride stress: A possible risk factor for chronic renal failure in the north-central province. Journal of National Science and Foundation. 2009;**37**(3):219-222

[25] Dharma-Wardana MWC. Chronic kidney disease of unknown etiology and the effect of multiple-ion interactions.

Environmental Geochemistry and Health. 2018;**40**(2):705-719. DOI: 10.1007/s10653-017-0017-4

[26] Valcke M, Levasseur ME, Soares da Silva A, et al. Pesticide exposures and chronic kidney disease of unknown etiology: An epidemiologic review. Environmental Health. 2017;**16**:49. DOI: 10.1186/s12940-017-0254-0

[27] Jayasumana C, Orantes C, Herrera R, Almaguer M, Lopez L, et al. Chronic interstitial nephritis in agricultural communities: a worldwide epidemic with social, occupational and environmental determinants. Nephrology Dialysis Transplantation. 2017;**32**(2):234-241. DOI: 10.1093/ndt/gfw346

[28] Singh S, Kumar V, Gill JPK, Datta S, Singh S, Dhaka V, et al. Herbicide glyphosate: Toxicity and microbial degradation. International Journal of Environmental Research and Public Health. 2020;**17**(20):7519. DOI: 10.3390/ijerph17207519

[29] Wang R, Chen J, Ding F, Zhang L, Wu X, Wan Y, et al. Renal tubular injury induced by glyphosate combined with hard water: The role of cytosolic phospholipase A2. Annals of Translational Medicine. 2021;**9**(2):130. DOI: 10.21037/atm-20-7739

[30] Dharmaratne RW. Fluoride in drinking water and diet: The causative factor of chronic kidney diseases in the north central province of Sri Lanka. Environmental Health and Preventive Medicine. 2015;**20**:237-242. DOI: 10.1007/s12199-015-0464-4

[31] Chandrajith R, Nanayakkara S, Itai K, Athuraliya TNC, Dissanayake CB, Abeysekera T, et al. Chronic kidney diseases of uncertain etiology (CKDue) in Sri Lanka: Geographic distribution and environmental implications. Environmental Geochemistry and Health. 2011;**33**:267-278

[32] Nanayakkara S, Senevirathna STMLD, Harada KH, Chandrajith R, Nanayakkara N, Koizumi A. The influence of fluoride on chronic kidney disease of uncertain aetiology (CKDu) in Sri Lanka. Chemosphere. 2020;**257**:127186. DOI: 10.1016/j.chemosphere.2020.127186

[33] Sansfica M, Young PHMTGA, Ishiga H. Factors controlling fluoride contents of groundwaterin north-central and northwestern Sri Lanka. Environmental Earth Science. 2011;**63**:1333-1342. DOI: 10.1007/s12665-010-0804-z

[34] Paranagama DGA, Bhuiyan MA, Jayasuriya N. Factors associated with chronic kidney disease of unknown aetiology (CKDu) in north central province of Sri Lanka: A comparative analysis of drinking water samples. Applied Water Science. 2018;**8**:151. DOI: 10.1007/s13201-018-0792-

[35] Moody GH, Southam JC, Buchan SA, Farmer JG. Aluminium leaching and fluoride. British Dental Journal. 1990;**169**(2):47-50. DOI: 10.1038/sj.bdj.4807270

[36] Bandara JM, Senevirathna DM, Dasanayake DM, Herath V, Bandara JM, Abeysekara T, et al. Chronic renal failure among farm families in cascade irrigation systems in Sri Lanka associated with elevated dietary cadmium levels in rice and freshwater fish (Tilapia). Environmental Geochemistry and Health. 2008;**30**(5):465-478. DOI: 10.1007/s10653-007-9129-6

[37] Mission Report. Chronic Kidney Disease of Uncertain Aetiology (CKDu), Sri Lanka. Geneva, Switzerland: Dr Shanthi Mendis. World Health Organization; 2011. Available from:

https://dokumen.tips/documents/who-full-report.html?page=1

[38] Herath S, Kawakami T, Nagasawa S, Serikawa Y, Motoyama A, Chaminda GGT, et al. Arsenic, cadmium, lead, and chromium in well water, rice, and human urine in Sri Lanka in relation to chronic kidney disease of unknown etiology. Journal of Water Health. 2018;**16**(25):212-222. DOI: 10.2166/wh.2018.070

[39] Stalin P, Purty AJ, Abraham G. Distribution and determinants of chronic kidney disease of unknown etiology: A brief overview. Indian Journal of Nephrology. 2020;**30**(4):241-244. DOI: 10.4103/ijn.IJN_313_18

[40] Desalegn B, Nanayakkara S, Harada KH, Hitomi T, Chandrajith R, Karunaratne U, et al. Mycotoxin detection in urine samples from patients with chronic kidney disease of uncertain etiology in Sri Lanka. Bulletin of Environmental Contamination and Toxicology. 2011;**87**(1):6-10. DOI: 10.1007/s00128-011-0301-4

[41] Aida T. Revisiting suicide rate during wartime: Evidence from the Sri Lankan civil war. PLoS ONE. 2020;**15**(10):e0240487. DOI: 10.1371/journal.pone.0240487

[42] Nanayakkara S, Senevirathna ST, Parahitiyawa NB, Abeysekera T, Chandrajith R, Ratnatunga N, et al. Whole-exome sequencing reveals genetic variants associated with chronic kidney disease characterized by tubulointerstitial damages in north central region, Sri Lanka. Environmental Health Preventive Medicine. 2015;**20**(5):354-359. DOI: 10.1007/s12199-015-0475-1

[43] Friedman DJ. Genes and environment in chronic kidney disease hotspots. Current Opinion in Nephrology and Hypertension. 2019;**28**(1):87-96. DOI: 10.1097/MNH.0000000000000470

[44] Educational Publications Department. Geography Grade 11. 2011

[45] Epidemiology Unit, Ministry of Health Sri Lanka. Screening Guidelines Chronic Kidney Disease Sri Lanka. 2017

[46] CKD Patients. Renal disease prevention unit. Provincial department of health service North- Central province [cited December 31, 2023]. 2023. Available from: https://healthdept.nc.gov.lk/renal-care-unit/

[47] Zhang S. Interpreting Sri Lanka's Organic Farming Failure. 2022. Available from: https://brownpoliticalreview.org/2022/11/sri-lankas-organic-farming-failure/#:~:text=First%20of%20all%2C%20Sri%20Lanka's,that%20transition%20within%20a%20year [Accessed: January 31, 2024]

Section 2

Dietetic Aspects and Diabetic Nephropathy

Chapter 5

Diet in Chronic Kidney Disease

Mohd. Aslam and Mohd. Hatif

Abstract

With the increasing incidence of CKD worldwide due to the causes involving multiple comorbidities such as hypertension, diabetes mellitus etc., CKD becomes a common disease throughout the world where nutrition plays an important role in the management of disease. Also, diet modification becomes necessary to control the intake of energy, proteins, fats, vitamins & minerals (Na^+, K^+, Ca^{+2} & phosphorus) in daily food ration which is quite a burdensome. Lack of adherence to dietetic recommendation contributes to low consumption of nutrients including energy, vitamins and minerals which can further lead to protein energy wasting (PEW) known as protein energy malnutrition (PEM) of CKD. Additionally, usage of patient-centred & cost-effective nutritional modifications and disease specific dietary changes may help in enhancing longevity and delaying the need of hemodialysis in millions of people across the world.

Keywords: diet, CKD, nutrition, protein energy wasting (PEW), protein, energy, carbohydrates, fats, minerals

1. Introduction

Chronic kidney disease is defined as evidence of structural or functional renal impairment for three or more months which is generally progressive and irreversibly affecting multiple metabolic pathways [1]. In CKD, alteration in protein & energy homeostasis, increase in protein catabolism, acid-base derangements and hormonal dysfunction occur which hinder normal growth and development of the patient. Chronic kidney disease can be categorized in stages according to GFR as described in **Figure 1**.

As chronic kidney disease progresses, accumulation of nitrogen containing products from dietary & intrinsic protein catabolism may blunt appetite. There are tendencies for negative nitrogen balance and loss of muscle mass which in consequence can lead to cachexia, exacerbated by coexisting conditions & fraility, particularly in adult patients. Hence, nutritional status of many patients often becomes disordered and protein energy wasting shows up ending with dietary adjustement requirements in CKD patients.

Nutritional therapy helps in managing various complications of CKD likewise uremia, electrolyte imbalance, acid-base imbalance, water & salt retention, mineral & bone disorders and failure to thrive. Again, it also helps in delaying or avoiding dialysis therapy. However, possible yet not proved, dietary therapy can also slow down the disease progression independent of uremia management. The symptoms of CKD vary according to the respective stages given in **Table 1**.

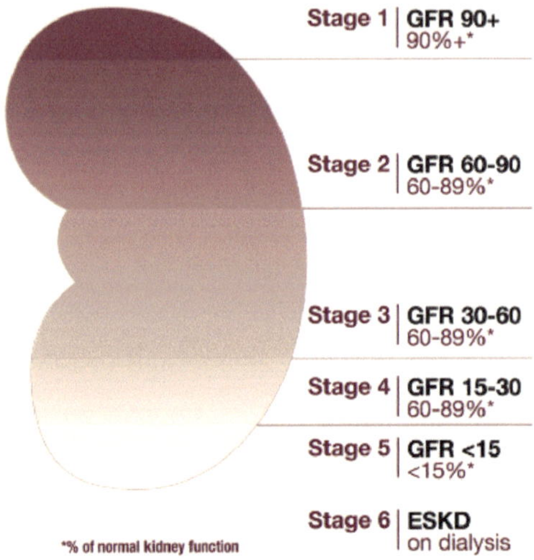

Figure 1.
Stages of chronic kidney disease (GFR in ml/min/1.73 m²).

2. General approach to dietary management

The widespread nutritional & metabolic alterations, high incidence of malnutrition and current evidence that dietary therapy retards the progression of CKD, indicates the critical aspect of nutritional therapy in CKD patients. There are mainly five goals of dietary management:

a. To maintain good nutritional status

b. To prevent or decrease uremic toxicity

c. To prevent or decrease metabolic disorders of renal failure

d. To reduce the risk of cardiovascular, cereberovascular and peripheral vascular diseases

e. To arrest or retard the progression of renal failure

Adherence to special diets is often difficult and frustating for patients & their families. This requires a team approach with support of family, doctor, dietician, nursing staff and whenever available social worker or psychiatrist, who can also help in improving the adherence capacity of patient to specific dietary changes.

3. Intrarenal hemodynamics

Dietary protein intake does not influence the level of systemic arterial blood pressure but intrarenal hemodynamics regularly respond to the changes in dietary protein intake and in return, protect against renal injury. Due to progressive loss of nephron in CKD, protein intake is a primary determinant of the degree of

Level of severity or risk	Normal kidney function (eGFR >60) and no proteinuria, but have CKD risk factors (diabetes, hypertension, or solitary kidney)	Mild to moderate CKD (eGFR 30–<60) without significant proteinuria (<0.3 g/day)	Advanced CKD (eGFR < 30) or any CKD with significant proteinuria (>0.3 g/day)	Transitioning to dialysis therapy with good reserve kidney functions including incremental dialysis preparation	Prevalent dialysis therapy, or any CKD stage with existing or imminent PEW
CKD stage	No CKD, or CKD stage 1 (eGFR >90) or stage 2 (eGFR 60–<90)	CKD Stage 3a (eGFR 45–<60) or 3b (eGFR 30–<45)	CKD stage 4 (eGFR 15–<30) or 5 (eGFR < 15)	Usually CKD Stage 5, although dialysis transition but it may happen at higher eGFR also	CKD stage 5, or any stage with PEW
Symptoms	At this stage, usually there are no symptoms related to kidney disease but patient may have symptoms related to the underlying conditions such as diabetes mellitus, polycystic kidneys or uncontrolled hypertension. Solitary kidney usually is not associated with any symptom unless ESRD develops.	Patient may have no symptom, but some may report fluid retention, e.g., oedema of dependent extremities upon upright position or facial oedema in the morning and shortness of breath. Urination changes such as nocturia (due to isosthenuria) may occur. Secondary hypertension may arise and result in symptoms if uncontrolled.	Worsening symptoms are often observed including more severe peripheral oedema and pulmonary symptoms due to fluid overload. Other symptoms include foamy urine, fatigue, pruritus, muscle cramps, restless extremities, altered mental status, sleep wake cycle disturbance, memory & concentration disorders, decreased taste & smell, diminished appetite, nausea & vomiting, growth retardation may occur in children.	Symptomatically deterioration and uremic complications may prompt transition to dialysis including decompensated heart failure, refractory hiccups, peripheral neuropathy, uremic encephalopathy, uremic bleed like gum bleeding or GI bleeding (due to platelet dysfunction), pericarditis, sexual dysfunction, amenorrhea, skeletal deformities. Weight loss, muscle wasting and symptoms related to electrolyte & mineral derangements such as hypocalcemia.	Additional symptoms related to dialysis treatment include post-dialysis light headedness & fatigue, worsening muscle wasting & weight loss, worsening cramps during dialysis treatment or with ultrafiltration and worsening cardiovascular symptoms such as palpitations or chest pain.

Table 1.
Clinical symptoms in different stages of chronic kidney disease (CKD).

functional & structural growth in remaining nephrons of remnant kidney. High protein intake stimulates the growth of cells (hypertrophy), exacerbate proteinuria and increases the weight of kidney while restricting protein intake prevents an increase in kidney size [2]. Likewise, both GFR and renal blood flow can be improved following an acute or chronic increase in dietary proteins. There is also an evidence, indicating a low protein diet lowers intraglomerular pressure by

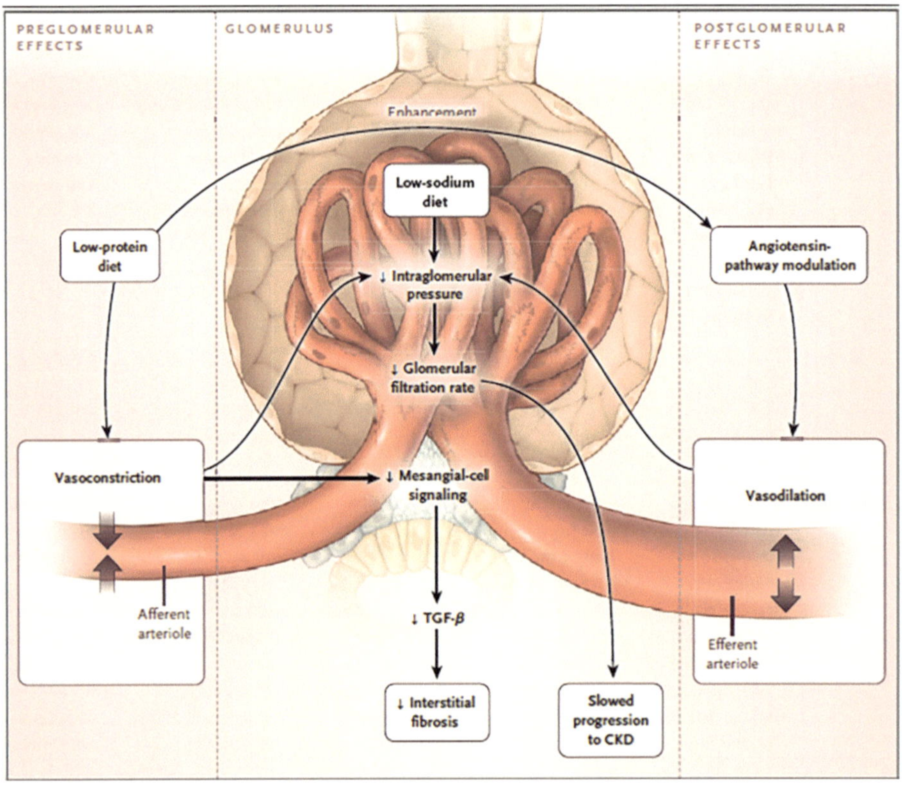

Figure 2.
Effects of low protein, low salt diet on afferent arteriole [3].

constricting the afferent arterioles and enhance the post glomerular effect of angiotensin pathway modulators that dilate efferent arterioles which further diminishes progressive renal injury (**Figure 2**) [3].

There are also various studies, stating the risks of toxicity from high protein diet which potentiates proteinuria and had both direct and indirect toxic effects on proximal tubular epithelial cells. Proteins also catabolize into some toxic intermediates (Indoxyl sulfate, phenylacetic acid) which contribute further in renal injury [4].

4. Assesment of nutritional status

Routine nutritional screening of CKD patients should be done at least biannually with the intent of identifying patients at risk of developing protein-energy wasting (PEW). Physical examination, body composition, anthropometric measurements and biochemical determinants are the components of nutritional assessment in CKD patients. Anthropometric measurements include practical, economical & non-invasive techniques that describe body mass, size & shape which is the most basic and an indirect method of assessing body composition. Likely, direct methods are bioelectrical impedance analysis (BIA), creatinine kinetics, near infrared and dual-energy X-ray absorptiometry (DEXA). These can be used in assessing body composition but they are expensive and cannot be used easily in different scenarios. DEXA is

Area	Assessments
Physical examination	Diet history, appetite assesement questionnaires, food diaries
Anthropometric measurements	Body weight, height, BMI Percentage weight change Skin fold thickness Midarm muscle circumference
Body composition	Neutron activation Near infrared reactance Bioelectrical impedence DEXA
Biochemical determinants	Serum electrolytes Serum proteins (albumin) Lipid profile (cholesterol) Creatinine index
Nutritional scoring systems	Subjective global assessment
Immunological assays	Hemogram (Lymphocyte counts) Delayed cutaneous hypersensitivity test
Functional test	Grip strength

Table 2.
Assessment tools for nutrition in CKD [5].

considered as a gold standard in assessing the body composition in patients of CKD but it is labour intensive, costly & an invasive method which can be easily altered by a number of factors such as hydration status in CKD (**Table 2**) [5].

There are limited evidences regarding the use of any one method over other for identifying patients who are at risk of protein-energy wasting (PEW).

4.1 Protein energy wasting (PEW)

Protein energy wasting is a syndrome consists of metabolic & nutritional abnormalities which often occur in CKD also called as PEM of CKD. It is associated with increased mortality and morbidity in CKD patients. There are various reasons for protein energy wasting like poor food intake, poor appetite, dietary restrictions, uremia induced alteration, chronic inflammation, metabolic acidosis & endocrine abnormalities which lead to hypermetabolism resulting in excess muscle & fat catabolism. Furthermore, contribution by low physical activity, fraility and hemodialysis precipitate in the development of PEW (**Figure 3**).

Serial assessment of CKD patients are done by using several scoring tools including Subjective Global Assesment (SGA), Malnutrition Inflammation Score (MIS), Geriartic Nutritional Risk Index (GNRI) and PEW Diagnostic Criteria.

PEW diagnostic criteria is used in making diagnosis of PEW, published by ISRNM, 2013, which is described in **Figure 4.**

From the above listed categories, at least three out of the four (3/4) (and at least one in each of the selected category) must be present in order to make the diagnosis of CKD related PEW. Each criteria should be fulfilled on at least three occasions, preferably 2–4 weeks apart [6].

The sequelae of PEW include malaise, fatigue, impaired wound healing, increased susceptibility to infections, increased cardiovascular disease risk and increased hospitalization & mortality rates (**Figure 5**).

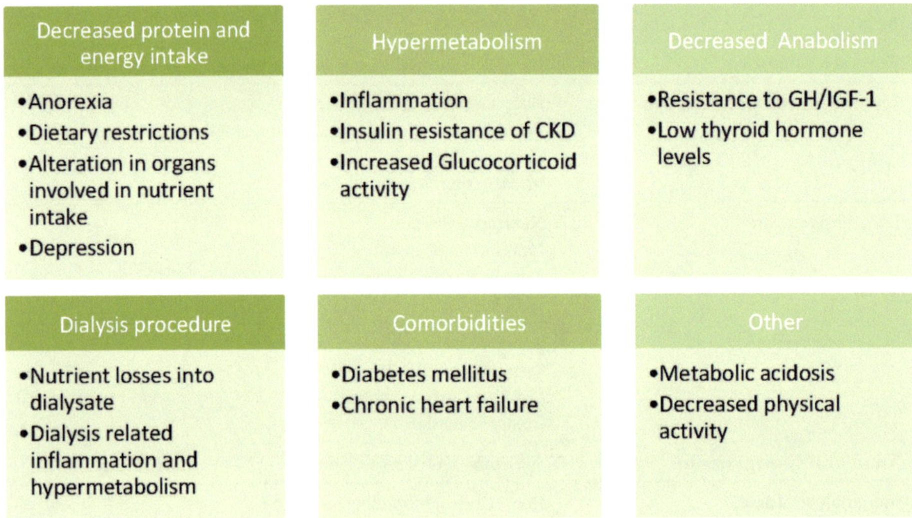

Figure 3.
Pathogenesis of PEW in CKD patients.

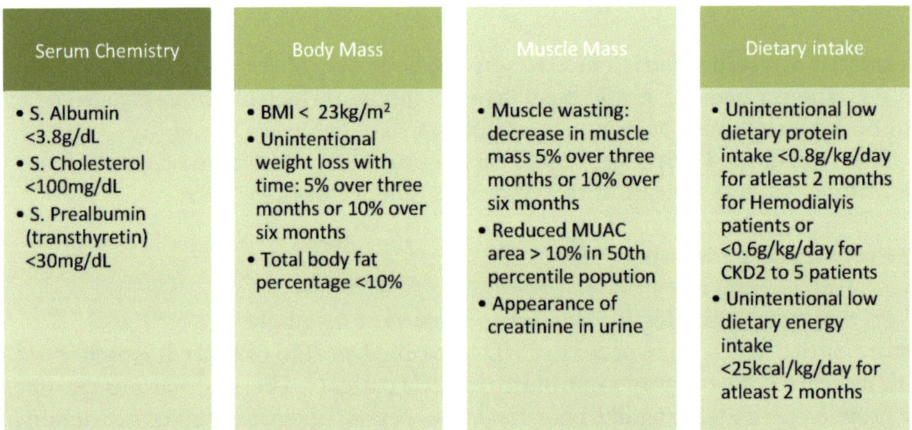

Figure 4.
PEW diagnostic criteria [6].

4.2 Tools for nutritional assessment

See **Figure 6**.

4.2.1 Patient interview and physical examination

Detailed history and physical examination have to be done in order to find out the risks of PEW. History has to be taken to find out the symptoms of nausea, vomiting, decreased appetite and recent changes in body weight. It is important to take history regarding uremic or non uremic causes and regarding the cause of CKD and PEW.

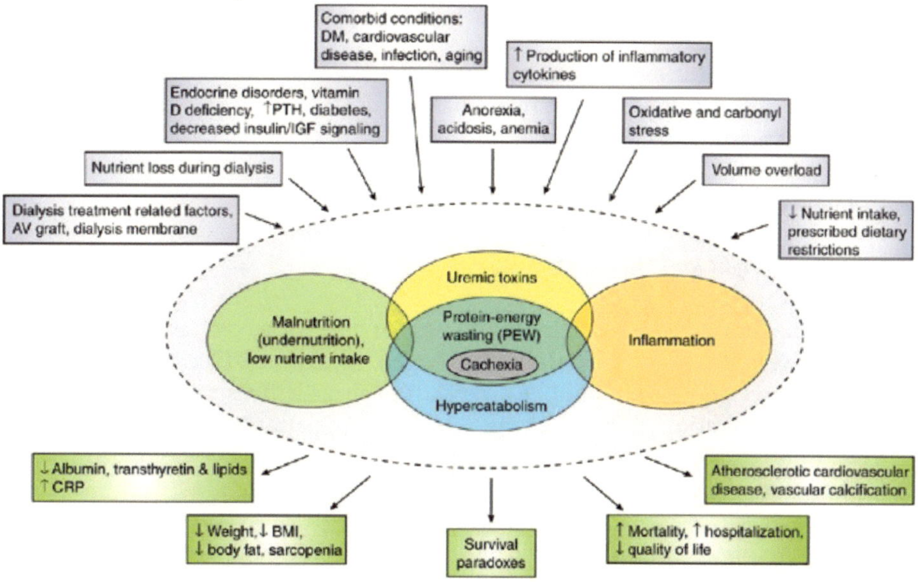

Figure 5.
Pathophysiology of PEW in CKD.

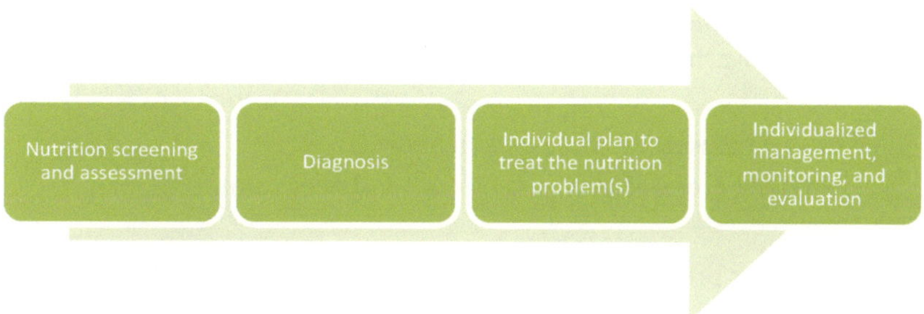

Figure 6.
Tools for nutritional assessment and management.

4.2.2 Assessment of food intake

24 hour food recall method can be used to know about the food intake on both dialysis and nondialysis days which should be performed twice in a year. Generally, food intake on dialysis days is about 20% lower as compared to non dialysis days. Assessment of food intake can also be done by using food frequency questionnaires.

4.2.3 Nutritional screening tools

Various tools can be used in screening of nutritional status of a CKD patient. The important ones are Malnutrition Universal Screening Tool (MUST), Mini Nutritional Assessment (MNA), Malnutrition Screening Tool (MST). The MST includes two questions; one regarding weight loss and other regarding appetite. If the score of these questions, when added together, comes out to be more than 2 then there is a high risk of developing malnutrition and PEW.

4.2.4 Nutritional assessment tools

When patient is screened positive for malnutrition then, further assessments have to be done by using various tools & methods to make the confirmed diagnosis of PEW. These assessments may include;

4.2.4.1 Body composition

4.2.4.1.1 Body weight and body mass index

Ideal or median standard weight should be measured and compared with the actual body weight. It is also important to compare ideal or median standard weight to the prior body weight. BMI should be used cautiously as it gives a poor estimate of fat mass and its distribution within the body, especially in patients with CKD.

4.2.4.1.2 Anthropometry

There are multiple anthropometric measurements which are used in assessing the patient nutrition, each with some advantages and disadvantages of their own. Waist to Hip Ratio (WHR) & Skinfold Thickness are used for classification of obesity in CKD patients which combinely show better results than BMI in various cross-sectional studies.

Skinfold thickness should be measured at the midpoint of biceps or triceps and can be related to mid-arm muscle circumference from the equation given below;

$$\begin{aligned}&\textit{Mid-arm}\text{ muscle circumference}(\text{MAMC})\\&=\textit{mid-arm}\text{ circumference}(cm)-\{3.14\times\text{triceps skinfold}(cm)\}\end{aligned} \tag{1}$$

Skinfold thickness provides an estimate of body fat whereas midarm circumference is useful in estimating muscle mass. If the values of either mid-arm circumference or triceps skinfold thickness is below the 25th percentile, patient is likely to be malnourished. In obese patients, skinfold thickness may not be accurate as most of the calipers have their upper limits that cannot accommodate high levels of adiposity.

4.2.4.1.3 Bioimpedance

When a constant alternating current is applied to the human body, there comes resistance & reactance by the body against the alternating current which is measured and termed as bioimpedance. The values of resistance & reactance are used in emperical equations which predict total-body water using resistance and total-body mass from the ratio of resistance to reactance or from the graph plotted between resistance & reactance as its geometrical derivative, the phase angle. In non-dialysed CKD patients or patients on peritoneal dialysis, there are insufficient studies & evidences suggesting the use of bioelectrical impedance in assessment of body composition but in CKD patients on MHD, bioimpedance preferably multi-frequency bioelectrical impedance (MF-BIA) can be used to assess body composition. It should be ideally performed after 30 minutes or more likely at the end of the hemodialysis session to allow redistribution of body fluids throughout the body [5].

4.2.4.1.4 Dual energy X-ray absorptiometry (DEXA)

In the beginning, DEXA used to measure the bone density but later it was adapted to quantify soft tissue composition of the body including muscle mass & fat. Now, DEXA is mainly used for research purposes as it is costlier than other methods. There is also no data relating DEXA that results in the outcomes of patients with advanced CKD but whenever feasible DEXA should be used in patients of CKD 1 to 5D and post-transplant patients because it is not easily influenced by hydration status of the patient and still remains the gold standard method for measuring body composition.

4.2.4.2 Biochemical parameters

4.2.4.2.1 Albumin

Albumin is a major circulating protein in the body that maintains the osmotic pressure and helps in transporting a variety of molecules. Serum albumin may be used as one of the best predicter of hospitalization & mortality in patients of CKD. Campbell et al. found that low albumin concentrations (<3.8 g/dL) were significantly associated with higher morbidity & mortality [5]. It also correlates with other nutritional assessment tools like bioimpedance and can be influenced easily by other inflammatory conditions & comorbidities.

4.2.4.2.2 24 hour urinary collection

It is performed to estimate dietary intake of proteins (urinary urea nitrogen), electrolytes (Na^+, K^+), creatinine clearance and proteinuria. It is also helpful in evaluating the adherence of patient to dietary recommendations which further, can be used in improving lack of adherence by suggesting the required changes in the diet. Excretion of protein end product as urea is easily measured and is often used to estimate adequacy of dialysis.

4.2.4.2.3 Acute phase reactants

There are various molecules & proteins that are related to the inflammation in CKD which may be increased or decreased according to the disease activity.

Serum prealbumin levels may be elevated because of interaction of prealbumin with retinol binding protein and decreased renal clearance. In hemodialysis patients, S. prealbumin <20 mg/dl are associated with increased risk of mortality, even in patients with normal albumin level. Also, fall in serum prealbumin over 6 months is independently associated with increase in mortality [7].

C-reactive protein (CRP) is a positive acute phase reactant which correlates negatively with Albumin and other proteins concentration in the body. When Albumin and Prealbumin levels are low, it is apt to check CRP levels which can help in revealing potential covert inflammation but its level is highly variable in ESRD patients.

In CKD patients there are also *decreased cholesterol* and *increased IL-6* levels which can also be used in assessment of nutritional status of the patient.

5. Nutritional guidelines

5.1 Macronutrients

5.1.1 Proteins

See **Figure** 7.

Proteins are responsible for adequate growth & development of children and maintenance of body structure in adults. Proteins are catabolized into urea and many other known & unknown compounds in the body. These compounds are cleared by the kidneys and get excreted in urine normally. When GFR starts to decline, these by-products get accumulated in the blood & different organs that progressively start getting affected leading to impaired organ functions as a consequence. Catabolized products of proteins are also responsible for a major fraction of kidney workload. Various studies and researches have confirmed the detrimental role of the renal hyperfiltration response associated with high protein intake in the kidneys causing further fall in GFR [8]. Therefore, in patients of CKD, reducing protein intake (0.55–0.6 g/kg/d) will reduce hyperfiltration which will have many beneficial effects like reduction in clinical symptoms, postpone the need of maintenance hemodialysis and decrease in mortality but on the other hand, reducing protein intake may also impair nutritional status in individuals who are at risk for PEW.

The quality of protein intake also matters. The rationale behind the use of proteins having branched chain amino acid is that during protein metabolism, these amino acids are deaminated by removal of an α-amino group leaving behind a carbon skeleton which can be recycled to form other amino acids and proteins or can be used in energy generation through the tricarboxylic acid cycle [9]. During protein catabolism, there is also generation of urea through the urea cycle. Hence, restricting dietary protein results in a proportional reduction in urea generation and use of ketoacids decreases the need of protein intake by providing the essential amino acids.

Protein intake can be classified according to relevant kidney disease conditions as suggested by MDRD study (**Table 3**) [3].

Protein intake in CKD can be determined according to CKD stages as described in **Figure 8.**

Factors such as providing adequate energy (30–35 kcal/kg/day), nutritional education and surveillance, may improve adherence to a low-protein diet [12].

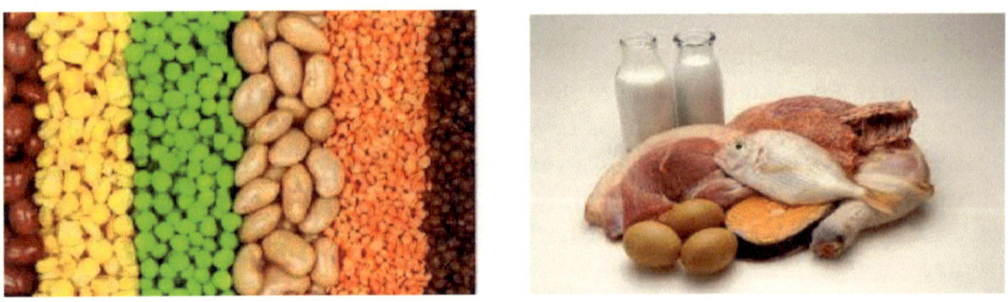

Figure 7.
Foods containing high amount of protein.

Dietary protein intake range	Daily protein intake grams per kg ideal body weight (g/kg/day)	Comment
Protein free diet	<0.30 g/kg/day	Not recommended in any person including CKD patients
Very low protein diet	0.3–0.6 g/kg/day	Have to be supplemented with essential amino acids, keto-acids or hydroxy-acids
Low-protein diet	0.6–0.8 g/kg/day	Recommended for advanced CKD (≥stage 3b or in patients having substantial proteinuria), usually no supplementation is needed until the diet contains at least 50% high biologic value proteins
Moderately low protein intake	0.8–1.0 g/kg/day	Recommended range for adults without CKD but have risk factors of CKD including diabetes mellitus, hypertension, solitary kidney (following nephrectomy), and polycystic kidneys
Moderate protein intake	1–1.2 g/kg/day	Recommended range for healthy adults without CKD or known risks of CKD, although most Americans eat higher DPI
Moderately high protein diet	1.2–1.5 g/kg/day	Recommended range for maintenance dialysis patients on conventional treatment, e.g. thrice weekly HD or daily PD, with minimal residual kidney function (urine urea clearance < 2 ml/min)
High to very high protein diet	>1.5 g/kg/day	Can be used for acute conditions such as hypercatabolic AKI, high grade burns, and severe PEW but over limited period of time

Table 3.
Ranges of dietary protein intake (DPI) according to kidney diseases [3].

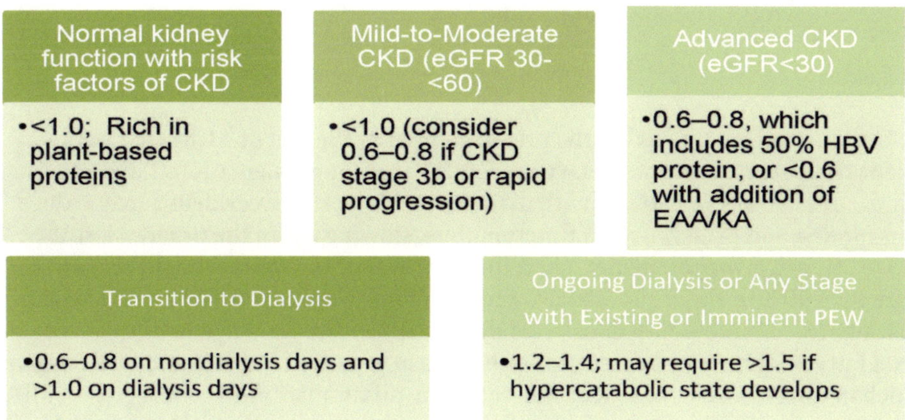

Figure 8.
Daily dietary protein intake in CKD patient (g/kg/day) [10, 11].

5.1.2 Energy

Adequate amount of energy is required in a diet of CKD patient in order to maintain desirable body mass, to limit gluconeogenesis and to prevent protein catabolism.

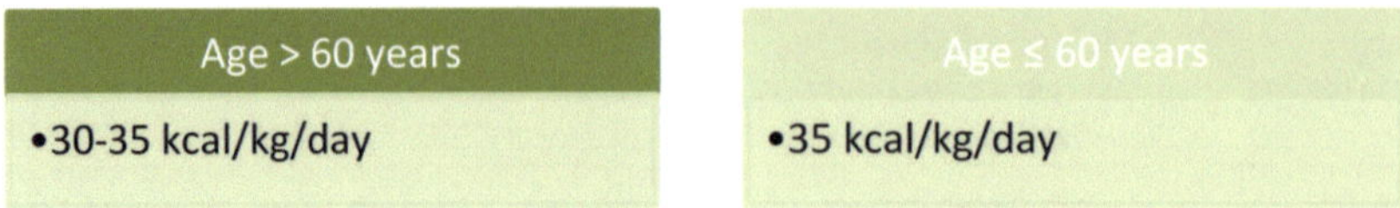
Age > 60 years
•30-35 kcal/kg/day
Age ≤ 60 years
•35 kcal/kg/day

Figure 9.
Daily energy requirement of CKD patients [13].

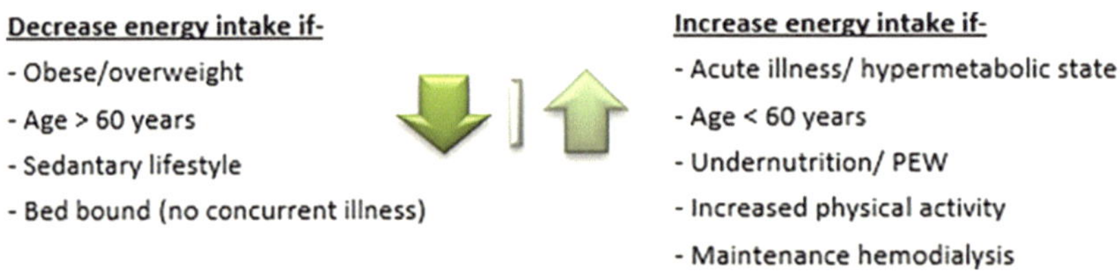
Decrease energy intake if-
- Obese/overweight
- Age > 60 years
- Sedantary lifestyle
- Bed bound (no concurrent illness)
Increase energy intake if-
- Acute illness/ hypermetabolic state
- Age < 60 years
- Undernutrition/ PEW
- Increased physical activity
- Maintenance hemodialysis

Figure 10.
Conditions requiring change in energy intake.

Number of factors are required to determine the energy intake in adults diagnosed with CKD. These include the age of patient, gender, weight, overall health status, level of physical activity, metabolic stressors and treatment goals.

According to KDOQI classification the energy requirement in CKD patients is defined as **Figure 9**.

Patients should be monitored routinely to assess the energy requirements and further, changes should be made in nutritional status if energy requirements are not met satisfactorily. Various conditions in which energy intake requires changes are described in **Figure 10.**

Protein and energy balance are the most important tasks in the prevention of PEW. In case of low protein diet, one should increase energy intake by using other sources of energy like carbohydrates and fats.

5.1.3 Fats

Unsaturated fatty acids are the preferred lipid in the diet of a CKD patient. A recent study suggested that dietary n − 3 fatty acid supplementation (flaxseed, canola, or olive oil) in patients with diabetes and hypertriglyceridemia may reduce albuminuria and preserve renal function thus, slowing down the progression of CKD [14]. In a low-protein diet, combined fats & carbohydrates should account for more than 90% of the required daily energy intake in order to avoid protein–energy wasting [15]. Total 25–35% of calories should come from fat. High intake of saturated fatty acid causes atherosclerotic changes in vessels of kidneys and other organs which in turn increase the risk of Malnutrition-Inflammation-Atherosclerosis (MIA) syndrome, leading to increased risk of cardiovascular deaths in CKD patients. Long-chain n − 3 PUFA helps both in reducing triglycerides & LDL cholesterol levels as well as in raising HDL levels.

The therapeutic goal in patients with CKD is to maintain the lipid levels in the range of;

- Low density lipid (LDL) < 100 mg/dl
- Fasting triglyceride levels < 500 mg/dl

With regards to diet composition, the usual recommendation is <7% saturated fat in diet, <10% of total calories should be derived from polyunsaturated fatty acids and <20% of total calories should come from monounsaturated fatty acids. Also, cholesterol should be <300 mg/day according to latest recommendations [14].

5.1.4 Carbohydrates and fibers

Carbohydrates are generally used in unrefined form and they make half of the usual daily energy intake which may be even higher in those having low protein diet. In patients with CKD, carbohydrate resources should also consist of fibers in higher amount (e.g., whole-wheat breads, multigrain cereal, oatmeal, mixed fruits & vegetables) which help in reducing absorption of dietary phosphorus and decrease generation of urea and creatinine as well [16]. Recommended intake of carbohydrates is *no lower than 130 g*. This ensures proper functioning of central nervous system & RBCs. Insufficient amount of carbohydrates in a diet can cause disruption in metabolism of fatty acids leading to accumulation of ketones and development of metabolic acidosis. Moreover, acidosis increases anorexia, promotes release of cortisol which enhances protein catabolism and also reduces the synthesis of albumin thus, intensifying malnutrition & loss of muscle mass. Hence, increased risks of PEW [17]. The right quality of sugar intake is also necessary as fructose increases obesity and risks of diabetes which further promote kidney damage. It is recommended that 50–60% of diet should contain carbohydrates that means 1000 kcal or 250 g of carbohydrates for a 2000 kcal diet. Fibers are another entity which is an important part of diet in patients of CKD. Diet of a vegetarian contains a good amount of fiber which helps in reducing dyslipidaemia by decreasing absorption of fat, K^+, uremic toxins etc. from GIT as they reduce gastrointestinal transit time. Fibers also generate favorable microbiome which helps in controlling uremic symptoms and slows down the disease progression. An amount of 20–30 g of fiber per day should be consumed which can help in reducing dyslipidaemia. In general, high fiber diets are also associated with lower cardiovascular mortality [18].

5.2 Micronutrients

Micronutrients in our daily food ration play an essential role in maintaining many metabolic functions and therefore should be present in adequate amount for which Daily Reference Intakes (DRIs) is made for each micronutrient. However, there is lack of evidence regarding appropriate intake of various micronutrients for people with CKD. The common reasons for deficiency of various micronutrients include insufficient dietary intake, dietary prescriptions which may limit vitamin-rich foods (particularly water-soluble vitamins), dialysis procedure, improper absorption of vitamins and certain medications & illnesses.

5.2.1 Sodium and fluids

Sodium is an extracellular cation responsible for fluid homeostasis in the body. In CKD patients, dietary sodium restriction is invariably recommended to control fluid retention and hypertension and to improve the cardiovascular risk profile. Patients with high sodium intake (>4 g/day) exhibit a strong relationship with hypertension while reduced sodium intake along with low protein and angiotensin modulation therapy result in decreased intraglomerular pressure which reduces proteinuria and slows down the disease progression. In CKD patients, the excretion of sodium is disturbed which can cause sodium retention and contribute in formation of oedema due to accumulation of water in tissues.

It is recommended that CKD patient should restrict sodium intake of <4 g/day while CKD patients with fluid retention and oedema should restrict sodium intake to <3 g/day. Excessive restriction of sodium of less than 1.5 g/day in CKD patients can cause hyponatremia and other adverse outcomes (**Figure 11**) [19].

$$\left[1\,\text{g salt} = 0.4\,\text{g}\,Na = 17\,meq\,Na^{+}\right] \quad (2)$$

CKD patients should limit fluid intake to less than 1.5 L/day due to isosthenuria, as excess of fluid intake can cause hyponatremia [19]. Additional fluid intake can be done if patient has residual renal function which is based on daily urine output & insensible fluid loss (**Figure 12**).

5.2.2 Potassium

Potassium is the main intracellular cation which plays an important role in mediating cellular electrophysiology, vascular functions, BP and neuromuscular functions. Abnormal potassium levels can cause muscular weakness, hypertension, ventricular arrhythmias and deaths. In CKD patients, the various mechanisms involved in the homeostasis of potassium (i.e. adrenergic system, insulin, aldosterone & urinary clearance) are impaired and hyperkalaemia can also be found in CKD patients on hemodialysis. There is a well-established association that states, high potassium with low sodium in diet can lower down the incidences of hypertension, stroke, nephrolithiasis and kidney diseases. In healthy adults and those at risk of kidney disease,

Mild to Moderate CKD	Advanced CKD/ any stage with hypertension or PEW/ Hemodialysis
•<4g/day	•<3g/day

Figure 11.
Daily requirement of Na^{+} intake in CKD patients [3].

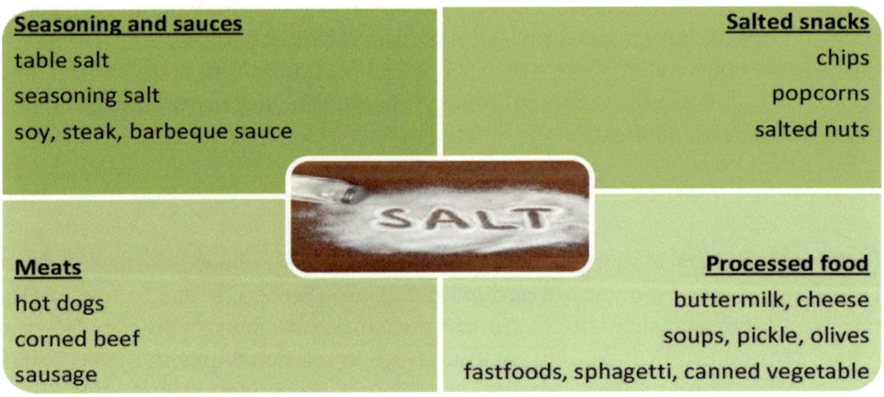
Seasoning and sauces
table salt
seasoning salt
soy, steak, barbeque sauce
Salted snacks
chips
popcorns
salted nuts
SALT
Meats
hot dogs
corned beef
sausage
Processed food
buttermilk, cheese
soups, pickle, olives
fastfoods, sphagetti, canned vegetable

Figure 12.
Foods to be avoided due to high sodium intake.

a relatively high daily potassium intake of 4.7 g (120 mmol) is recommended [20]. Although, in patients with kidney diseases, a higher dietary potassium intake may be associated with a higher risk of poor kidney disease progression. According to various epidemiologic studies, both moderately low plasma potassium levels (<4.0 mmol/liter) and high levels (>5.5 mmol/liter) are associated with rapid kidney disease progression. In patients of advanced kidney disease and hyperkalaemia, it is advised to restrict dietary potassium intake to less than 3 g/day (<77 mmol/day) but excessive dietary restrictions can expose the patient to more atherogenic diets and worsen constipation which may actually result in higher gut potassium absorption [21]. A reduction in the consumption of potassium is usually achieved by limiting or excluding potassium rich fruits and vegetables from daily food ration (DFR) (**Figure 13**).

During restriction of potassium intake, intake of fresh fruits & vegetables with high fiber should not be compromised. Potassium content in vegetables & fruits can be lowered by soaking them in water for 2–4 hours, a process called *leaching* and also boiling can be used otherwise. Both the techniques are associated with reduced food taste and palatability which can be improved by using aromatic herbs (**Figures 14** and **15**).

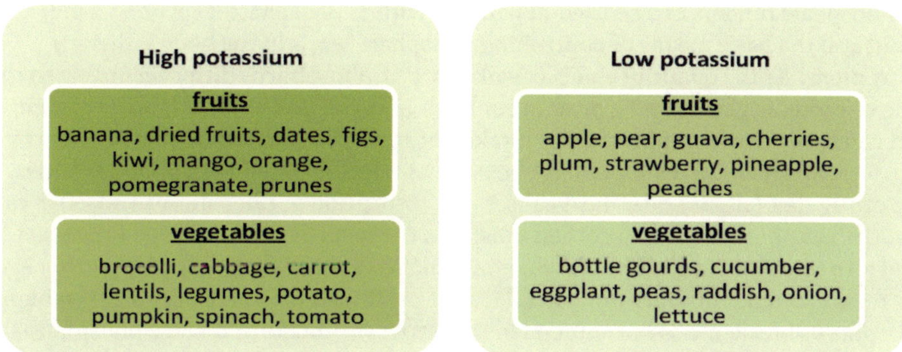

Figure 13.
Potassium containing foods.

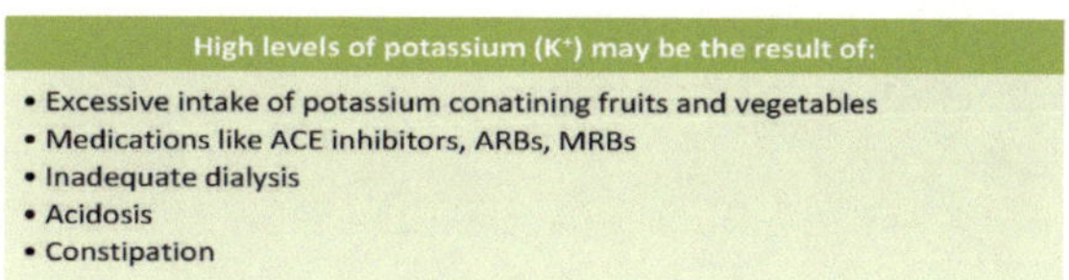

Figure 14.
Conditions associated with increased level of K^+.

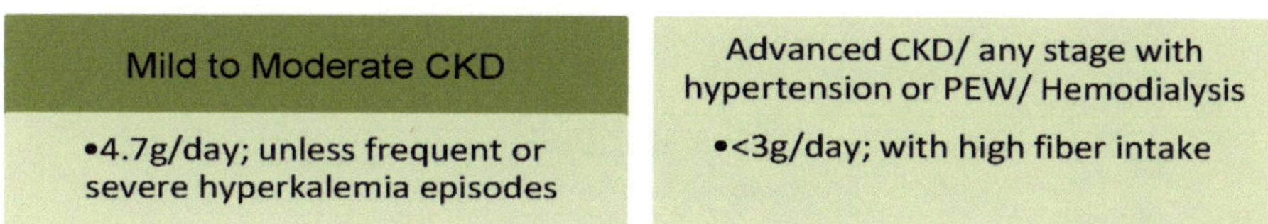

Figure 15.
Daily requirement of K^+ intake in CKD patients [3].

5.2.3 Phosphorus

Phosphorus is an essential nutrient required for bone growth & mineralization as well as for regulation of acid-base homeostasis. Phosphorus is present in most foods both as a natural component and added as an approved ingredient during food processing. It is necessary to control dietary levels of phosphorus in order to avoid hyperphosphatemia. In CKD patients, there is an abnormal renal function which causes excess phosphorus in the body resulting in hyperphosphatemia leading to disorders of bone and mineral metabolism. Hyperphosphatemia which can cause complications is infrequently seen in early stages of CKD (stage 1–3) as there are high levels of both parathyroid hormone as well as fibroblast growth factor 23 (FGF-23) in blood and tissues, promoting urinary phosphorus excretion. Patients at stage 5 of chronic kidney disease, receiving dialysis therapy or who are at increased risk for protein–energy wasting, there are low levels of vit D_3 & calcium which cause elevated parathyroid hormone and FGF-23 but due to poor renal function phosphorus is not excreted therefore, it gets accumulated in body and causes vascular calcification, renal bone diseases, left ventricular hypertrophy and accelerated progression of kidney disease from vascular & tubulointerstitial injury [22].

Phosphate binders can be used in patients with S. Phosphate level of >5.5 mg/dl but still the basic means of controlling phosphate levels in the body is dietary restrictions. As the quantity and bioavailability of phosphorus differ according to the type of protein (generally 1 g protein contains 13 mg of phosphorus), a low protein diet can easily decrease phosphorus intake but stringent restriction of phosphate by restricting protein intake should not be done as it is associated with poor outcomes. Use of veg diet (fibers) over meat causes low absorption of phosphorus (30–50% vs. 50–70%) as phosphorus is absorbed mostly in the form of phytates [23]. Processed food also contains readily absorbable inorganic phosphorus and this phosphorus is not mentioned on the Nutrition Facts label of processed food results in an even higher phosphorus burden. It is recommended to restrict the intake of dietary phosphorus to less than 800 mg/day (26 mmol/day) from all sources for patients with moderate to advanced kidney diseases (**Figures 16** and **17**).

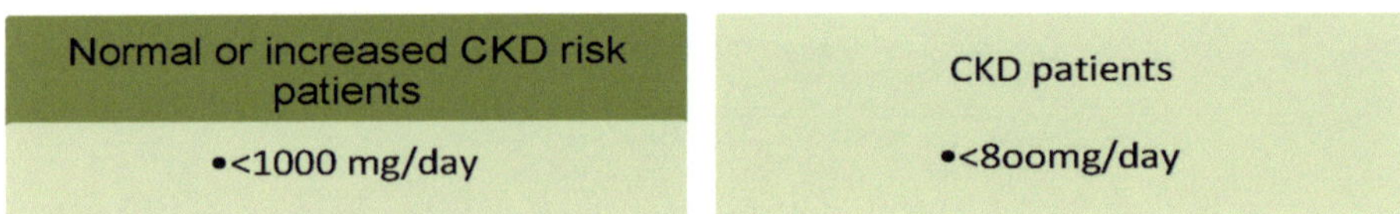
Normal or increased CKD risk patients
•<1000 mg/day
CKD patients
•<8oomg/day

Figure 16.
Daily requirement of phosphorus in CKD patients [11].

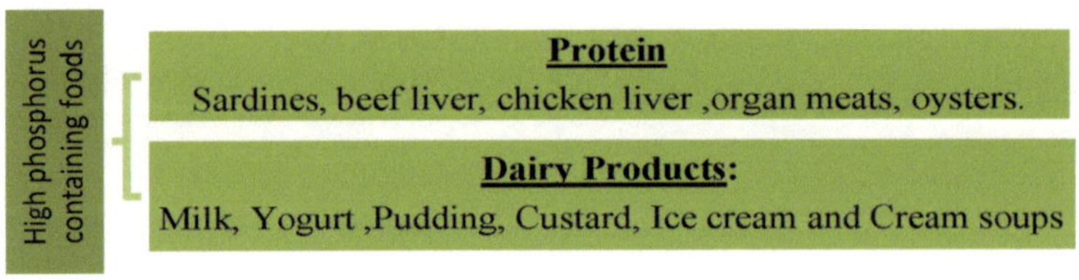

Figure 17.
High phosphorus containing foods.

5.2.4 Calcium

Calcium plays an important role in maintenance of bone health, nerve impulse conduction, muscle contraction, blood coagulation, hormone secretion and intercellular adhesions. Approximately all of total body calcium is found in the bones and a small proportion is present in the extracellular and intracellular spaces. Calcium balance is tightly regulated by calciotropic hormones (vitD_3 and PTH) at multiple levels in the body such as absorption from the intestine, reabsorption from kidneys and exchange from bones. Calcium balance in CKD is poorly understood, its concentration is maintained in normal ranges until very late in CKD where it decreases but slightly. It is due to decrease in vitD_3 in CKD patients which causes decrease in gut absorption of calcium and causes secondary hyperparathyroidism resulting in decreased calcium excretion in urine and increased calcium release from bone in the form of ionized calcium and may cause positive calcium balance responsible for extraosseous calcium deposition like in blood vessels which can increase risks of cardiovascular mortality in CKD patients [24].

According to many studies, calcium intake in normal adults without kidney disease is 1000–1300 mg/day (25–32 mmol/day) while in CKD stage 3 or 4, 800–1000 mg of elemental calcium per day (20–25 mmol/day) in the diet will result in a stable calcium balance in the body. In patients with ongoing dialysis or any stage with existing PEW, <800 mg of elemental calcium per day from all sources should suffice and prevents extraosseous complications (**Figure 18**) [25].

The total intake of elemental calcium (including both dietary and elemental calcium) should not exceed more than 2000 mg/day.

5.2.5 Other minerals

5.2.5.1 Iron

Iron deficiency is common among CKD patients due to various reasons which can further result in iron deficiency anemia. People with advanced kidney disease and those on hemodialysis lose iron from digestive tract due to frequent bleeding episodes caused by uraemia, frequent blood investigations and hemodialysis itself. In CKD patients, iron deficiency can be absolute iron deficiency, in which patients have severely reduced or absent iron stores or functional iron deficiency, in which patients have adequate iron stores but iron cannot be incorporated into erythroid precursors due to increased levels of hepcidin leading to anemia of chronic disease. Iron deficiency criteria is different among CKD patients as compared to normal people. Among CKD patients, absolute iron deficiency is defined as transferrin saturation (TSAT) ≤20% and serum ferritin concentration ≤100 ng/mL (in pre dialysis and peritoneal dialysis patients) or ≤200 ng/mL (in hemodialysis patients).

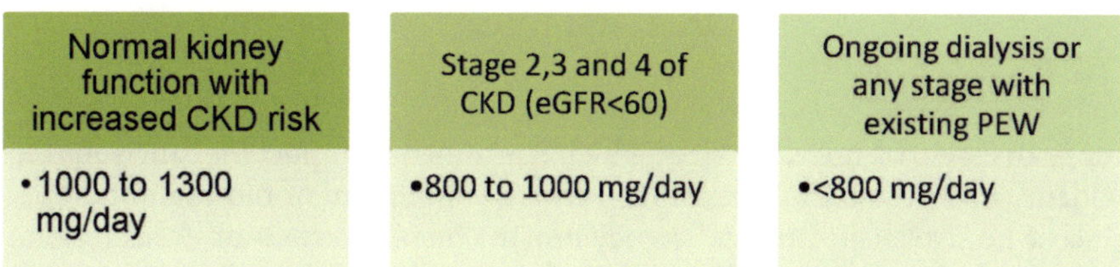

Figure 18.
Daily calcium requirements in CKD [3].

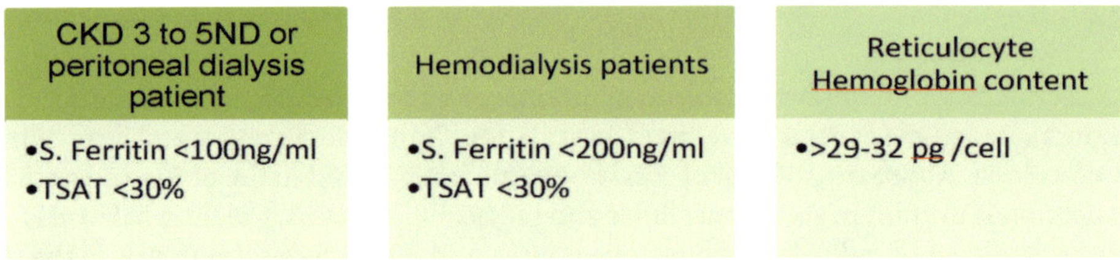

Figure 19.
Goals for iron stores in CKD patients [5].

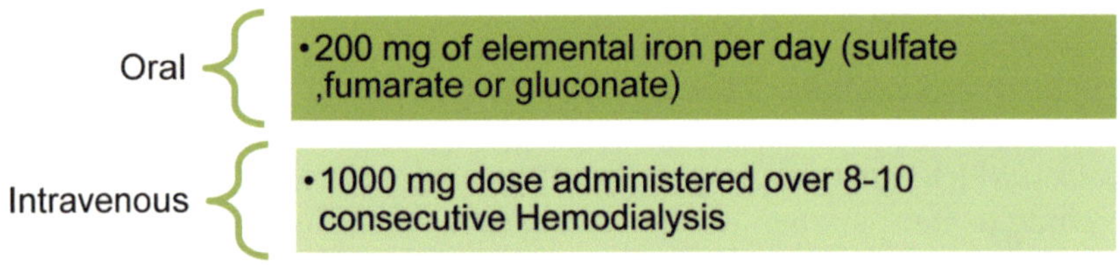

Figure 20.
Different routes and doses of iron administration.

Serum ferritin is an acute phase reactant and is generally higher in CKD patients due to diffuse inflammation which characterizes advanced kidney disease and hemodialysis [25]. Intravenous iron supplementation is the preferred method for advanced CKD patients while both Intravenous or oral iron is recommended for patients with moderate CKD. Oral iron has generally poor efficacy in hemodialysis patients but in Peritoneal Dialysis it is much more convenient to use (**Figure 19**).

Iron can be administered via different routes and doses as described in **Figure 20** [26].

5.2.5.2 Magnesium

The main source of magnesium in daily food ration are grain products, milk & milk products and potatoes. As these also contain phosphorus and potassium, patients with chronic kidney disease are often seen not taking these diets. Hypomagnesemia is also caused by tubular dysfunction and interstitial fibrosis which impair tubular magnesium reabsorption. Deficiency of magnesium is related to early tubular cell death and inflammation induced by phosphate load thus, increase the risk of end-stage kidney disease along with high-serum phosphate levels. It also has a capacity to inhibit the calcification of vascular smooth muscle cells induced by phosphate thus, retarding the progression of coronary artery calcification among non-dialysis CKD patients. Patients on hemodialysis with mild hypermagnesemia exhibit low mortality rate. Approximately, 200–300 mg/day of magnesium intake should be there.

5.2.5.3 Zinc

Zinc is an essential micronutrient which has multiple important functions like antioxidant, anti-inflammatory effects, forms a component of bio-membranes and glucose homeostasis. Zinc deficiency impairs insulin formation & secretion, decreased leptin levels and present as loss of appetite, taste disturbances, growth inhibition & slower wound healing. Deficiency is attributed to low intake of the bio element with the diet and increasing renal failure. Intake should be based on recommendations for the general population that is 8 mg/day for women and 11 mg/day for men [5]. There are no specific changes recommended as no such strong relation has been found in between zinc and CKD.

5.2.5.4 Selenium

Selenium is a trace element that has known antioxidant properties and acts as a cofactor for various antioxidant enzymes like glutathione peroxidase. CKD patients have low levels of selenium which can result in increased oxidative injury and inflammation. There are also some studies which suggest that low levels of selenium may be associated with increased risk of mortality in advanced kidney diseases and patients on MHD, especially, from infections [27]. There is not enough evidence to make recommendation of selenium supplementation for malnutrition-inflammation syndrome in MHD patients. The current Recommended Dietary Allowance (RDA) for selenium is 55 mcg/d for women and men [5].

5.2.5.5 Copper

Copper is also a micronutrient which is mainly found in vegetables, cereals, meat, fish, poultry, & legumes. The recommended daily intake of copper for adults is 900 mcg/day but the average daily intake is between 1 mg and 1.6 mg. Absorption of copper from the gut and the amount present in the diet are responsible for maintaining adequate levels of copper in the body both of these which are reduced in patients on hemodialysis causing deficiency of copper.

5.3 Vitamins

5.3.1 Fat soluble vitamin

Proper level of fat-soluble vitamins (A, E, D and K) in a diet is important due to their antioxidative role in the body. Fat soluble vitamins are not removed by dialysis and therefore should not be supplemented unless their deficiency is noted.

5.3.1.1 Vitamin D

Vitamin D2 (ergocalciferol) and vitamin D3 (cholecalciferol) are recognized as a pro hormones. There are two sources of vitamin D as it can be absorbed from gut and can also be synthesized by the human skin through the action of sunlight [28].

The functions of vitamin D include regulation of calcium & phosphorus in the body and various other potential pleiotropic effects like on immune, cardiovascular & neurological systems. Some studies also suggests that vitamin D has some antineoplastic activity. A number of factors and conditions contribute to decreased vitamin D levels in patients with CKD like dietary restrictions, loss of vitamin D binding protein (DBP) during hemodialysis, reduced sun light exposure, aging, diabetes mellitus and obesity. In some studies, vitamin D analogues have been associated with decreased proteinuria along with reversal of renal osteodystrophy [29]. Again, many studies suggest that there is a significant decline in PTH levels via supplementation of cholecalciferol or ergocalciferol in CKD patients including renal transplant recipients. Hydroxylated vitamin D agents may be needed in addition to native vitamin D to control progressive secondary hyperparathyroidism. Vitamin D2 (ergocalciferol) and

Vit. D - 15 to 29 ng/ml	Vit. D < 15 ng/ml
•50,000 IU/Month for 6 months of vit. D_2 or D_3	•50,000 IU/week for 2-3 months then 50,000 IU/monthly of vit. D_2 or D_3

Figure 21.
Daily requirement of Vit. D in CKD patients [5].

vitamin D3 (cholecalciferol) have to be given in patients according to vit. D levels in blood. Vitamin D supplementation (cholecalciferol or ergocalciferol) may be given to the CKD patients with low serum vitamin D levels (<30 ng/ml) (**Figure 21**).

5.3.1.2 Vitamin A and E

It is reasonable to not routinely supplement vitamin A or E because of the potential for vitamin toxicity. Optimal serum levels of vitamin E are not defined for CKD patients. There is an increased risk of impaired platelet aggregation and haemorrhagic stroke in cases of high doses of vitamin E supplementation because vitamin E interacts with both anticoagulant & antiplatelet drugs. Therefore, its supplementation has to be avoided in CKD patients who are already receiving these medications [30]. High levels of vitamin A can cause anemia and lipid abnormalities. Oral doses ≥400 IU of vitamin E is not recommended without at least intermittent monitoring of serum vitamin E levels [5].

5.3.1.3 Vitamin K

Vitamin K acts as a cofactor for enzyme gamma-glutamyl carboxylase which is needed for carboxylation of various proteins like coagulation factors (II, VII, IX and X). Deficiency of these factors can lead to impaired blood clotting and increased risk of bleeding. Vitamin K also participates in normal bone formation and structure by helping in the carboxylation of proteins which control calcium deposition in bones (e.g., osteocalcin). Matrix G1a protein (MGP) is a vitamin K-dependent protein produced by vascular smooth muscle cells which inhibits vascular calcification and atherosclerotic plaque calcification in vessels [5].

There are two classes of vitamin K, phylloquinone (vitamin K1) from plant products and menaquinones (vitamin K2) from animal/dairy products both of which are responsible for vitamin K activity. In CKD patients on antibiotics, vitamin K deficiency can be aggravated by multiple factors and can lead to elevated prothrombin time due to increasing age, thrombocytopenia & platelet dysfunction, high serum urea & creatinine and low serum albumin concentrations [31]. Vitamin K supplementation may return prothrombin time to normal in such patients. The recommended dietary vitamin K intake for CKD patients is not defined, it is similar to general population. Vitamin K supplementation is needed in hemodialysis patients on antibiotics or those who are not eating as they have low serum vitamin K.

5.3.2 Water soluble vitamins

Water soluble vitamins like vitamin B complex, folate and vitamin C are removed by dialysis and should be supplemented in diet. High flux dialysis removes greater quantity of water-soluble vitamins. Despite water solubility of *thiamine* (*B1*), *riboflavin* (*B2*), *pantothenic acid* (*B5*) and *biotin* (*B7*) plasma concentrations of these vitamins are not usually decreased in patients undergoing MHD. It can be due to counterbalance of loss of these vitamins in hemodialysis and no excretion in urine.

Niacin (*B3*) concentrations have been reported to be low in patients undergoing MHD and therefore supplemented in dose of 7.5 mg/day.

Pyridoxine (*B6*) many studies show the deficiency of vit. B6 concentration in many patients undergoing hemodialysis. B6 supplements improve various parameters of immune function in MHD patients including lymphoblast formation. Treatment with pyridoxine decreases plasma homocysteine levels and plasma oxalate concentrations. 5 mg of pyridoxine HCl is supplemented in non-dialysed patients of CKD 1 to 5 and 10 mg in patients undergoing MHD.

Folic acid is also decreased in patients undergoing MHD which along with B12 deficiency can also causes anemia and hyperhomocysteinemia. Dietary folic acid requirements are increased in CKD 4 and 5 during the time when they commence erythropoietin therapy. Supplementation of folic acid 1 mg/day is adequate in patients of CKD and if hyperhomocysteinemia is present it is given in the doses of 5–15 mg/day.

Vitamin B12 deficiency is uncommon in patients of CKD because its daily requirement is less (3 μg/day) and it is also protein bound in plasma hence, poorly dialysed. Therefore, no extra supplementation is needed in patients of CKD.

Ascorbic acid (*vitamin C*) acts as an antioxidant but in patients with high iron stores or transferrin, it releases catalytic iron from ferritin and drives cycle of repetitive reduction of ferric to ferrous forms which causes free radical injury [31]. Vitamin C is also decreased in patients undergoing MHD as foods rich in vitamin C also contains good amount of potassium such as citrus fruits and juices and are restricted for these patients. Clinical signs suggestive of mild scurvy has been found in many patients undergoing MHD. Kang et al. [32] reports that intravenous vitamin C (500 mg IV in each hemodialysis session for 3 months) is effective in erythropoietin resistant normoferritinemic anemia thus, helps in reducing cost, risk of exposure and adverse effects of erythropoietin & iron [33]. CKD patients at any stage and post-transplant are at risk of Vitamin C deficiency. For these patients, vitamin C is supplemented at a dose of 90 mg/day for men and 75 mg/day for women. Higher doses of Vitamin C supplementation (500 mg daily) also require caution as they have been shown to increase serum oxalate levels and can deposit in tissues in the form of oxalate crystals. Therefore, it should be supplemented in short term to avoid oxalosis [32, 34].

6. Discussion

As enlightened in this chapter, significance of putting forward the need for daily food requirements of various nutrients to control the progression of CKD. Also as discussed, the importance of sticking to those requisites which as a consequence prevent the development of malnutrition via rapid fall in GFR and delay the need for MHD. Therefore, is it of utmost priority that patients must comply to follow the specific diet as recommended. Except for, such high magnitude of changes in the diet for a patient, especially CKD stage 3–5 & patient on MHD is so overwhelming that if presented at once, the patient could become demoralized and lose his motivation. So, the goal is to prioritize the dietary modifications which mainly address the control of protein, energy, sodium, potassium, phosphorus & magnesium with a need to supplement calcium & vitamins along the diet. Patients with lipid disorders have higher risks of developing cardiovascular adverse events. It is better to use statins & fibrates initially to overcome the challenge so that, the patient can focus on other aspects of necessary alternations in diet. If the patient complies well with former dietary modifications, latter nutrients can be explored more intensively with the patient. A good compliance to low protein diet can be regularly assessed by using urinary nitrogen excretion. It is recommended that patients with CKD should be more careful while considering their food preferences. They must opt for consultation from a registered dietician to work on diet plans specific to the patient provided his resources. One can also find a registered dietician specialized in kidney diseases through 'Academy of Nutrition and Dietetics'. Here, the dietician counsels the patient regarding the required changes in diet according to medical & health goals. Another approach is 'Medical Nutrition Therapy' (MNT) in which management of kidney diseases is done through a tailored nutritional plan. Dietician plays an important role in providing the right diet plan & maintaining the compliance of patient to the dietary modifications. Patient can improve their dietary intake by discussing with their dietician about the food they prefer. As a result, a better & healthy diet plan can be made with patient preferences which will help to overcome challenges. In order to maximize the compliance to the diet, patient should visit the dietician regularly to make a 7-day meal plan & modifications in their diet monthly. A patient should never consider to make any change in the recommended diet without consulting their dietician. While attending both physician & dietician, it will consume patient's great amount of time from their daily routine which can hinder the process & patient's compliance. Thereby, it is needed that a specialized physician dedicated to both treat & suggest dietetic programs in a single setting made possible. It will ultimately help to improve the clinical outcomes & quality of life of patients with CKD. There are certain government organizations & limited private insurance companies that pay for certain number of visits to dietician and one can also opt for MNT with dietician under his insurance. Many research publications such as Modification of Diet in Renal Disease (MDRD), National Kidney Foundation, National Institute of Diabetes & Digestive & Kidney Diseases (NIDDK) and KDOQI Clinical Practice Guideline for Nutrition in CKD show the importance of dietary modifications in the management of CKD. These guidelines help both physician and dietician to modify diet of patients with CKD in accordance to their stage of disease. Further researches can be done to discover the importance of dietary modification in the management of CKD that in future will help us to improve the quality of life and clinical outcomes in CKD patients.

7. Conclusion

Approximately 10% of the adult population worldwide has chronic kidney disease. Given the high incidence & prevalence of chronic kidney disease and considering the exceptionally high costs and burden of maintenance dialysis therapy & kidney transplantation, an urgent need for patient-centred and cost-effective alternative disease management strategies such as nutritional interventions with disease-specific dietary ranges may help in increasing longevity and can prolong the dialysis-free interval for millions of people.

Acknowledgements

I'd like to express my gratitude to Almighty and everyone who helped me completing this chapter. Furthermore, I would also like to thank my guide and teacher (Prof. Mohd. Aslam) who helped me throughout the chapter with his valuable guidance and ideas. I would like to give my special thanks to my parents & my friends because without their special suggestions and support, it would not have been easy to complete this project.

Glossary

BIA	bioelectrical impedance analysis
Ca^{+2}	calcium
CKD	chronic kidney disease
DXA	dual-energy X-ray absorptiometry
ESRD	end stage renal disease
EAA	essential amino acids
MHD	maintenance hemodialysis
PD	peritoneal dialysis
HBV	high biological value
KA	keto acids
K^+	potassium
Na^+	sodium
PEM	protein energy malnutrition
PEW	protein energy wasting
FGF-23	fibroblast growth factor 23

Author details

Mohd. Aslam and Mohd. Hatif*
Jawaharlal Nehru Medical College and Hospital, AMU, Aligarh, India

*Address all correspondence to: hatifmohd@gmail.com

References

[1] Levey AS, de Jong PE, Coresh J, et al. The definition, classification, and prognosis of chronic kidney disease: A KDIGO controversies conference report. Kidney International. 2011;**80**:17-28

[2] Cirillo M, Lombardi C, Chiricone D, De Santo NG, Zanchetti A, Bilancio G. Protein intake and kidney function in the middle-age population: Contrast between cross-sectional and longitudinal data. Nephrology, Dialysis, Transplantation. 2014;**29**:1733-1740

[3] Ingelfinger JR, Kalantar-Zadeh K, Fouque D. Nutritional management of chronic kidney disease. New England Journal of Medicine. 2017;**377**:1765-1776. DOI: 10.1056/NEJMra1700312

[4] Niwa T, Ise M. Indoxyl sulphate, a circulating uremic toxin, stimulates the progression of glomerular sclerosis. The Journal of Laboratory and Clinical Medicine. 1994;**124**:96

[5] Ikizler TA, Burrowes JD, Byham-Gray LD, Campbell KL, Carrero J-J, Chan W, et al. KDOQI Clinical Practice Guideline for Nutrition in CKD: 2020 update. DOI: 10.1053/j.ajkd.2020.05.006

[6] Fouque D, Kalanter Zadeh K, Kopple J, et al. A proposed nomenclature and diagnostic criteria for PEW in acute and chronic kidney disease. Kidney International. 2008;**73**:391-398

[7] Fiedler R, Jehle PM, Osten B, Dorligschaw O, Girndt M. Clinical nutrition scores are superior for the prognosis of haemodialysis patients compared to lab markers and bioelectrical impedance. Nephrology, Dialysis, Transplantation. 2009;**24**(12):3812-3817

[8] Wrone EM, Carnethon MR, Palaniappan L, Fortmann SP. Association of dietary protein intake and microalbuminuria in healthy adults: Third National Health and Nutrition Examination Survey. American Journal of Kidney Diseases. 2003;**41**:580-587

[9] Garlick and Reeds. Metabolism of Carbon Skeleton of Amino Acid Chain Protein and Amino Acids. Washington, DC: National Academy of Sciences, Institute of Medicine, Food and Nutrition Board; 2005. DOI: 10.17226/10490

[10] Garneata L, Stancu A, Dragomir D, Stefan G, Mircescu G. Ketoanalogue-supplemented vegetarian very low-protein diet and CKD progression. Journal of the American Society of Nephrology. 2016;**27**:2164-2176

[11] Ko GJ, Obi Y, Tortorici AR, Kalantar-Zadeh K. Dietary protein intake and chronic kidney disease. Current Opinion in Clinical Nutrition and Metabolic Care. 2017;**20**:77-85

[12] Wu HL, Sung JM, Kao MD, Wang MC, Tseng CC, Chen ST. Nonprotein calorie supplement improves adherence to low protein diet and exerts beneficial responses on renal function in chronic kidney disease. Journal of Renal Nutrition. 2013;**23**:271-276

[13] KDOQI Clinical Practice Guideline for Nutrition in CKD:2020 Update. 2020;**76**(3, Suppl. 1):S1-S107

[14] Han E, Yun Y, Kim G, et al. Effects of omega-3 fatty acid supplementation on diabetic nephropathy progression in patients with diabetes and hypertriglyceridemia. PLoS One. 2016;**11**(5):e0154683

[15] Kovesdy CP, Kopple JD, Kalantar-Zadeh K. Management of protein-energy wasting in non-dialysis-dependent chronic kidney disease: Reconciling low protein intake with nutritional therapy. The American Journal of Clinical Nutrition. 2013;**97**:1163-1177

[16] Chiavaroli L, Mirrahimi A, Sievenpiper JL, Jenkins DJ, Darling PB. Dietary fiber effects in chronic kidney disease: A systematic review and meta-analysis of controlled feeding trials. European Journal of Clinical Nutrition. 2015;**69**:761-768

[17] Kraut JA, Madias NE. Metabolic acidosis of CKD: An update. American Journal of Kidney Diseases. 2016;**67**(2):307-317

[18] Sumida K, Molnar MZ, Potukuchi PK, et al. Constipation and incident CKD. Journal of the American Society of Nephrology. 2017;**28**:1248-1258

[19] Kovesdy CP, Lott EH, Lu JL, et al. Hyponatremia, hypernatremia, and mortality in patients with chronic kidney disease with and without congestive heart failure. Circulation. 2012;**125**:677-684

[20] Smith et al., 1992, Sebastian et al., 1994, Morris et al., 1999b. Water, Potassium, Sodium, Chloride, and Sulfate. Washington, DC: National Academy of Sciences, Institute of Medicine, Food and Nutrition Board; 2004. DOI: 10.17226/10925

[21] St-Jules DE, Goldfarb DS, Sevick MA. Nutrient non-equivalence: Does restricting high-potassium plant foods help to prevent hyperkalemia in hemodialysis patients. Journal of Renal Nutrition. 2016;**26**:282-287

[22] Faul C, Amaral AP, Oskouei B, et al. FGF23 induces left ventricular hypertrophy. The Journal of Clinical Investigation. 2011;**121**:4393-4408

[23] Moorthi RN, Armstrong CL, Janda K, Ponsler-Sipes K, Asplin JR, Moe SM. The effect of a diet containing 70% protein from plants on mineral metabolism and musculoskeletal health in chronic kidney disease. American Journal of Nephrology. 2014;**40**:582-591

[24] Bushinsky DA. Clinical application of calcium modeling in patients with chronic kidney disease. Nephrology, Dialysis, Transplantation. 2012;**27**:10-13

[25] Spiegel DM, Brady K. Calcium balance in normal individuals and in patients with chronic kidney disease on low- and high-calcium diets. Kidney International. 2012;**81**:1116-1122

[26] Nissenson AR. Achieving target hematocrit in dialysis patients: New concepts in iron management. American Journal of Kidney Diseases. 1997;**30**:307

[27] Fujishima Y, Ohsawa M, Itai K, et al. Serum selenium levels are inversely associated with death risk among hemodialysis patients. Nephrology, Dialysis, Transplantation. 2011;**26**(10):3331-3338

[28] Holick MF. Vitamin D deficiency. The New England Journal of Medicine. 2007;**357**(3):266-281

[29] de Zeeuw D, Agarwal R, Amdahl M, et al. Selective vitamin D receptor activation with paricalcitol for reduction of albuminuria in patients with type 2 diabetes (VITAL study): A randomised controlled trial. Lancet. 2010;**376**:1543-1551

[30] Miller ER 3rd, Pastor-Barriuso R, Dalal D, Riemersma RA, Appel LJ,

Guallar E. Meta-analysis: High-dosage vitamin E supplementation may increase all-cause mortality. Annals of Internal Medicine. 2005;**142**(1):37-46

[31] Williams KJ, Bax RP, Brown H, Machin SJ. Antibiotic treatment and associated prolonged prothrombin time. Journal of Clinical Pathology. 1991;**44**(9):738-741

[32] Kang DW, Ahn CY, Ryu BK, Shin BC, Chung JH, Lim HL. The Effect of Intravenous Ascorbic Acid in Hemodialysis Patients with Normoferritinemic Anemia. DOI: 10.1016/j.krcp.2012.01.002

[33] Herbert V et al. Vitamin C-driven free radical generation from iron. American Institue of Nutrition. 1996

[34] Singer RF. Vitamin C supplementation in kidney failure: Effect on uraemic symptoms. Nephrology, Dialysis, Transplantation. 2011;**26**(2):614-620

Chapter 6

Adipose Tissue as Risk Factor for Kidney Disease

Venera Berisha-Muharremi and Blerim Mujaj

Abstract

Obesity remains the leading risk factor for increased risk of acute kidney diseases and increased risk for progression to chronic kidney disease. Accumulation of excess adipose tissue in various body compartments is an underpinning characteristic of obesity. In the human body, adipose tissue in the body is mainly stored as subcutaneous adipose tissue (SAT) and visceral adipose tissue (VAT). Adipose tissue is biologically active and may interact with metabolic processes. Excess adipose tissue accumulation may be pathogenic through adverse endocrinologic or immunologic activity, and metabolic changes affect kidney function by decreasing the glomerular filtration rate (eGFR). Estimation of GFR is mainly based on serum biomarkers such as serum creatinine and or cystatin C. Adipocytes release cystatin C in a time-dependent manner and are not associated with serum creatinine. Pathophysiological mechanisms linking adipose tissue and cystatin C in humans remain unknown, and potential crosstalk mechanisms related to adipose tissue and kidney diseases remain scarce. In the clinical context, assessment of kidney function is based on the eGFR calculation based on serum biomarkers measurement, and whether other inflammatory parameters may help to explore the pathophysiological link or mechanism between adipose tissue and kidney function through biomarkers exploration remains unknown. This chapter aims to provide further insights into the mechanisms that link adipose tissue and kidney crosstalk by exploring kidney function biomarkers.

Keywords: adipose tissue, visceral adipose tissue, subcutaneous adipose tissue, creatinine, cystatin C, eGFR, kidney function, kidney disease

1. Introduction

Obesity, coupled with other co-morbidities such as diabetes and hypertension, remains the leading risk factor for increased risk of acute kidney diseases and increased risk for progression to chronic kidney disease, which leads to premature mortality globally [1]. The main characteristic of obesity is an accumulation of excess adipose tissue in various body compartments. However, adipose tissue in the body is mainly stored as subcutaneous adipose tissue (SAT), which plays a vital role in thermoregulation, and as visceral adipose tissue (VAT), which has a higher degree of metabolic activity [2]. Biological functions of adipose tissue may interact with metabolic processes, excessive mass alone may be pathogenic through adverse endocrinologic or immunologic activity, and metabolic changes may affect kidney

IntechOpen

function [3]. Glomerular filtration rate (GFR) [4] is the most helpful index for kidney function assessment [4], and reduction of GFR may indicate acute kidney injury (AKI) or chronic kidney disease (CKD) [5]. GFR estimation is mainly based on serum biomarkers such as serum creatinine and or cystatin C [6–8]. Both biomarkers are widely used in clinical practice; however, relatively imprecise GFR estimates remain, which may affect both acute and chronic illness, and such imprecision may result in the misclassification of patients with an estimated GFR of less than 60 ml per min/1.73 m^3 that might lead to unnecessary therapeutic interventions. When using serum creatinine as a biomarker for GFR estimation, several factors, such as muscle mass, physical activity, and protein-rich food intake, may influence its levels. Cystatin C is considered an alternative to serum creatinine for estimating GFR and is less affected than serum creatinine. As non-glycosylated protein synthesized and released by most nucleated cells, filtered by glomerulus, and catabolized by proximal tubules, cystatin C may also be influenced by inflammation, thyroid gland, tobacco use, thyroid disease, and obesity. Adipose tissue, defined as VAT and SAT, has been reported to be associated with impaired kidney function when cystatin C was used for GFR determination [9–11]. Adipocytes release cystatin C in a time-dependent manner. Yet, pathophysiological mechanisms linking adipose tissue and cystatin C in humans remain unknown, and potential mechanisms related to adipose tissue and kidney diseases remain scarce. Despite the clinical assessment of kidney function being based on the eGFR calculation—based on biomarkers measurement, the pathophysiological link or mechanism between adipose tissue and kidney function and biomarkers remains unknown. This chapter aims to provide further insights into the mechanisms that link adipose tissue and kidney disease by exploring kidney function biomarkers.

2. Adipose tissue and kidney disease

Adipocites and preadipocites are components of the adipose tissue, which ordinarily cellular part consists of 50% fat cells and the remaining 50% as preadipocites containing vascular stroma, endothelial cells, fibroblasts and macrophages [2, 12]. The main functions of adipose tissue are thermogenesis and energy storage; therefore, there are two distinct types of adipose tissue in the human body: subcutaneous adipose tissue (SAT), which plays an essential role in thermogenesis with lesser metabolic activity or function, and visceral adipose tissue (VAT) as fat storage mainly located in the abdominal region that is metabolically active, with increased vascularization, sympathetic innervation, and β3-adrenergic receptors. Factors such as adipocyte apoptosis, preadipocyte differentiation, lipolysis, lipogenesis, adipocyte receptors, cytokines, and adipokine secretion differ for fat depots. Although SAT is thought to be protective, even excessive subcutaneous adipose tissue may become pathogenic [13]. Under the conditions of obesity, the accumulation of fatty tissue in the abdominal cavity and surrounding internal organs is characterized as visceral adipose tissue, which later is pathogenically implicated in endocrine functions [3]. VAT is represented as a significant risk factor for cardio-metabolic diseases, which later affect kidney function. Loss or damage of nephrons, the kidney's functional units, is the underpinning pathophysiological pathway of kidney diseases. Within nephrons, podocytes are the fundamental cells of the glomerular barrier that selectively filter a range of macromolecules [14]. Podocytes are highly specialized and terminally differentiated cells that no longer can divide; therefore, malfunctioning or damaged podocytes can no longer be replaced. Thus, podocytes undergo hypertrophy to maintain the glomerular barrier integrity [15, 16].

Further, podocyte dysfunction or damage causes albuminuria, and increased albumin leak through the glomerular membrane promotes a pro-inflammatory reaction that can lead to interstitial inflammation and damage, leading to nephron dysfunction [17]. Adipose tissue, obesity-related glomeruli-associated damage is a concept proposed to describe the kidney function changes followed by glomerulopathy with podocyte damage and loss, glomerulosclerosis as a complex of kidney abnormality that includes glomerulomegaly and mesangial expansion, increased blood flow and hyper-filtration [18, 19]. A cascade of kidney function changes is directly linked to adipose tissue in early stages with reduced eGFR, followed by albuminuria, podocyte dysfunction, glomerulomegaly, glomerulosclerosis, and tubulointerstitial fibrosis. However, obesity with excess VAT, along with other risk factors or co-morbidities, indirectly contributes to kidney disease with a complex cascade of pathophysiological changes in the human body, such as increased systemic inflammation, the release of adipokines and cytokines, lipotoxicity, insulin resistance, renin-angiotensin system (RAAS) activation, and hypertension. Given that a decrease in GFR may indicate acute kidney injury (AKI) or chronic kidney disease (CKD), estimation of GFR based on biomarkers such as serum creatinine and cystatin C is the most reliable assessment of kidney function, the most widely used clinical practice.

Nevertheless, differences in tissue origin and production rates of compounds exist. The creatinine muscular source is well documented [4, 20], whereas the contribution of different organs in the production of circulating levels of cystatin C has been reported to be associated with VAT [10, 21], and similar findings have been found in an animal study [22]. Yet, mechanisms that relate adipose tissue and cystatin C remain unknown.

3. Adipose tissue pathophysiological mechanisms and kidney disease

3.1 Adipose tissue storage and kidney disease

The pathogenesis of the adipose tissue is significantly influenced by metabolic hormonal [23, 24] processes on how the adipose tissue is stored, through hypertrophy or hyperplasia, but also depending on the compartment of the human body where the adipose tissue is stored [2, 25, 26]. In positive caloric balance, metabolic processes or genetic factors determine how the adipose tissue is stored, whether adipocytes respond through hypertrophy or hyperplasia. In the adipogenic process, some factors may have different effects on adipocytes and non-adipocytes upon differentiation (adipocyte maturity and lipogenesis) or proliferation (new adipocytes from non-adipocytes) [27]. These two processes are driven by hormones such as glucocorticoids, angiotensinogen, and angiotensin II, which are closely related to metabolic disorders and fat storage deterioration [28–30]. The resulting hypertrophy compared to hyperplasia of fatty tissue, especially VAT versus SAT, in practical terms, has clinical implications given that it triggers adipose tissue paracrine activity, function, or dysfunction that promotes metabolic disorders such as type 2 diabetes mellitus, hypertension, and dyslipidemia [31, 32] and later affects the kidney function also. Alternatively, the location of adipose tissue is another crucial factor in whether fat depots have pathogenic potential. VAT, more accumulated in the abdomen or so-called abdominal adiposity, produces bioactive molecules and metabolism compared to less metabolically active SAT, which is accumulated and distributed in peripheral subcutaneous tissue.

Similarly, peri-organ adipose tissue, through metabolic activities, including the release of inflammatory factors and or lipolysis, may have a pathogenic impact on target organs, including kidneys [33]. In this context, accumulation of adipose tissue in the abdominal cavity and surrounding organs, mainly as VAT, represents a major risk for metabolic disorders leading to kidney diseases, indirectly and directly, as inner and/ or outer ectopic VAT exacerbates the normal function of kidneys, similar liver steatosis, and within a period of time leading to chronic kidney disease. This condition is more recognizable as fatty kidney disease [34] and is characterized by the spread accumulation of adipose tissue and reduced function in general. Previously, a study assessing the role of intra-renal adipose tissue reported a strong association with VAT, hypertension, albuminuria, and decreased kidney function [35, 36]. Nevertheless, as suggested above, the intra- and extra-renal VAT interplays bidirectionally, negatively impacting kidney function by directly affecting kidney hemodynamics. These changes lead to hyper-filtration, albuminuria, and, finally, impairment in GFR rate due to glomerulosclerosis, indirectly exacerbating various metabolic and inflammatory risk factors [35].

3.2 Adipose tissue, inflammation, and kidney disease

Adipocytes, in particular VAT adipocytes, are metabolically active cells that produce hormonal factors such as adiponectin, leptin, resistin, and visfatin but also inflammatory factors such as cytokines, including tumor necrosis factor (TNF)-a, interleukin (IL)-6, and interleukin (IL)1β [3, 37]. Although adipocytes and cytokines are intimately involved in developing inflammation, free fatty acid release, oxidative stress, and insulin resistance, their mechanism of action is poorly understood. However, their action is attributed to activating the rennin-angiotensin-aldosterone system (RAAS) [38]. Adiponectin receptors are widespread within glomeruli cells, including podocytes [39], and in mice, reduced adiponectin levels have negatively impacted podocyte function [40]. Free fatty acid, glucose metabolism, and insulin resistance are inversely associated with adiponectin levels, and in obesity, adiponectin levels are decreased, whereas leptin levels are increased [41].

On the other hand, leptin increases proportionally with adipose tissue and is key to energy balance and homeostasis regulator [42]. While leptin levels in CKD increase, it is unclear whether such levels are related to decreased GFR, given that leptin is principally cleared via the kidneys. Leptin and adiponectin have established effects on kidneys [3], and adiponectin may be produced locally within the kidneys rather than acting in an autocrine inter-organ crosstalk manner by exerting metabolic and inflammatory functions. In addition to triggering the sympathetic nervous system, leptin promotes hypertension [43], whereas adipokine accelerates the oxidation of free fatty acids, oxidative stress, and secretion of cytokines [44, 45]. Further, adipose tissue is a known source of pro-inflammatory cytokines, which are secreted systemically within and around the kidney and contribute to an inflammatory state of the kidney. The crosstalk in the adipose-renal axis is crucial for response to kidney injury as well as normal kidney function. Secretions of cytokines, tumor necrosis factor (TNF)-a, interleukin (IL)-6, and interleukin (IL)1β, and other cytokines result in the response of macrophages and other immune cells [46]. Engagement of immune cells may initiate or worsen the inflammatory environment of kidneys, inter-organ, and around, contributing to immune system dysfunction and low-grade inflammation, which later may progress into chronic kidney disease [47].

Furthermore, adipose tissue macrophages significantly produce other inflammatory factors, including cathepsin S, macrophage inhibitory factor, nerve growth factor, and inducible nitric oxide synthase (iNOS) [48, 49]. Noteworthy, other adipose tissue inflammatory factors reactants that potentially are pathogenic in the acute phase of kidney injuries, such as c-reactive protein, plasminogen activator inhibitor 1 (PAI-1), proteins of the complement system, chemotactic adipokines, prostaglandins and reduced anti-inflammatory factors [50–53]. Ion functional disturbances in the kidney tubule, leading to renal fibrosis, may be due to abnormal inflammatory processes in general but also due to the involvement of plasminogen activator inhibitor 1 (PAI-1), illustrating the complex cascade of the pathogenesis of CKD.

3.3 RAAS activation, insulin resistance, and kidney disease

The renin-angiotensin-aldosterone system (RAAS) is a critical system influenced by the VAT and excess circulating insulin. VAT, whether located in the abdomen cavity or the kidney, in inter-organ, due to endocrine activity, increases intra-renal pressure and RAAS activation [54]. RAAS is inappropriate under conditions of obesity and insulin resistance, and individuals with excess VAT show increased plasma renin activity, angiotensinogen, and circulating aldosterone [55]. The RAAS activation leads to sodium retention in tubules, contributing to systemic and intra-renal hypertension and impacting renal blood flow, perfusion, and intra-glomerular hypertension [56]. Consequently, related stress is imposed on renal vasculature glomerular cells and podocytes, and eventually, there is a decline in kidney function [57]. Alternatively, insulin resistance plays a vital role in kidney damage development. Predominantly, insulin resistance is driven mainly by pro-inflammatory cytokines released principally by VAT. Circulating cytokines affect insulin signaling [58], modulating the glomerular filtration barrier and podocyte function [59]. Animal and in vitro studies documented that insulin increased the glomerular permeability to albumin [60]; in clinical practice, conditions with hyperinsulinemia and hyperglycemia are associated with albuminuria [61]. Also, insulin resistance has been shown to promote the progression of renal fibrosis [62].

3.4 Thyroid, adipose tissue, and kidney disease

The thyroid gland drives metabolic processes in the human body, and hormonal alternations are associated with kidney diseases [63]. Thyroid function, including thyroid function disease, can affect kidney function and progression to CKD. In patients with CKD and end-stage kidney disease, low-free triiodothyronine (fT3) is present, and these patients are prone to hypothyroidism [64]. However, when renal function declines, thyroid hormone alternations occur, and thyroid stimulation hormone (TSH) rises, with or without reduced free thyroxine (fT4) and low fT3 [65]. Interestingly, kidney function improves in patients with thyroid hormone supplementation. The hormonal alternations of the thyroid are traditionally interpreted in the context of kidney dysfunction within the concept of non-thyroid disease. However, the possibility that disturbances may arise due to other pathways or diseases is seldom discussed. Despite sufficient evidence linking thyroid and kidney disease, the causality and directionality of the association still need to be made clear. Also, there is insufficient evidence about impaired thyroid function's role in patients with preserved or moderated reduced estimated glomerular filtration rate (eGFR) [63]. At the same time, thyroid hormones are determinants of energy expenditure and contribute to regulating appetite and releasing cytokines from adipose tissue, which inform the central nervous system (CNS) on energy storage [66]. In other words, there is a crosstalk between the thyroid and adipose tissue in the human body, and the thyroid drives mechanisms to localize and store adipose tissue [66].

On the contrary, data report that thyroid hormones did not directly cause CKD progression in the general population after 20 years of follow-up [67]. Nevertheless, there is an insufficient understanding of disease or kidney function impairment in the absence of thyroid disorders, and given the crucial role of thyroid hormones on adipose tissue, an under-recognized triangle mechanism may explain this relationship compared to the individual relationship between thyroid and kidney or adipose tissue and kidney only. From a physiological standpoint, kidney function assessment is based on GFR estimation based on serum creatinine and/or cystatin C. The first biomarker is related to thyroid and muscle metabolism. In contrast, the second biomarker, thyroid, has a significant impact on cystatin C [68] levels, which at the same time is released by adipose tissue, suggesting that an underlying biological plausible axis exists between thyroid, adipose tissue, and kidney disease crosstalk mechanism that needs further exploration. Recent animal studies indicated that triiodothyronine (T3) increases the production of cystatin C in adipocytes [22]. Similar findings have been reported from a study in the German population, free of kidney diseases, that VAT has been associated with serum cystatin C and reduced eGFR. In addition, triiodothyronine (T3) has been found to promote adipose tissue hyperplasia and mediate adipocyte proliferation [69]. Tracing further the effect of triiodothyronine (T3) on adipocytes suggests that it influences adipocyte hyperplasia. In contrast, later, the adipocytes, through the release of cytokines, impair the conversion of thyroxine (fT4) into triiodothyronine (T3).

4. Conclusion

Summarizing this chapter, a cascade of changes and mechanisms involved in interactions of adipose tissue and kidney function, we discussed the basis of this inter-organ crosstalk, which includes adipose tissue storage, inflammation RAAS

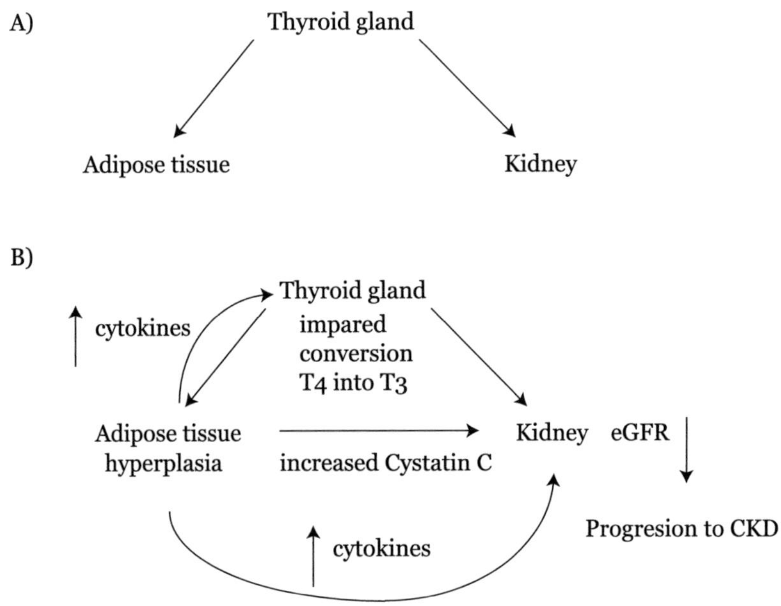

Figure 1.
Crosstalk between adipose tissue and kidney function, physiology (panel A) and pathophysiological mechanisms (panel B).

activation, and insulin sensitivity. However, characterizing further fundamental cellular changes at the level of adipocytes and affected changes of the microenvironment of adipocytes through the influence of thyroid function builds the new mechanistic infrastructure of inter-organ crosstalk between three key players: thyroid, adipose tissue, and kidney. Further elaboration of serum cystatin C levels may help identify relevant pathways to new axis thyroid-adipose tissue-kidney dysfunction into progression to kidney disease (**Figure 1**).

Author contributions

All authors contributed equally to this chapter. Conceptualization, V.B.M, B.M, writing—original draft preparation, V.B.M, B.M; writing—review and editing, V.B.M, B.M; visualization, V.B.M, B.M. All authors have read and agreed to the published version of the chapter.

Conflict of interest

The authors declare no conflict of interest.

Author details

Venera Berisha-Muharremi[1] and Blerim Mujaj[2,3*]

1 Faculty of Medicine, Department of Endocrinology University Clinical Center, University of Prishtina, Prishtina, Kosovo

2 Research Association Alliance Institute for the Promotion of Preventive Medicine (APPREMED), Mechelen, Belgium

3 General Practice, Huisartsenpraktijk, Aalst, Belgium

*Address all correspondence to: blerim.mujaj@gmail.com

References

[1] Whaley-Connell A, Sowers JR. Obesity and kidney disease: From population to basic science and the search for new therapeutic targets. Kidney International. 2017;**92**(2):313-323

[2] Bays HE, González-Campoy JM, Bray GA, Kitabchi AE, Bergman DA, Schorr AB, et al. Pathogenic potential of adipose tissue and metabolic consequences of adipocyte hypertrophy and increased visceral adiposity. Expert Review of Cardiovascular Therapy. 2008;**6**(3):343-368

[3] Zhu Q, Scherer PE. Immunologic and endocrine functions of adipose tissue: Implications for kidney disease. Nature Reviews Nephrology. 2018;**14**(2):105-120

[4] Levey AS, Stevens LA, Schmid CH, Zhang YL, Castro AF 3rd, Feldman HI, et al. CKD-EPI (Chronic Kidney Disease Epidemiology Collaboration). A new equation to estimate glomerular filtration rate. Annals of Internal Medicine. 2009;**150**(9):604-612. DOI: 10.7326/0003-4819-150-9-200905050-00006. Erratum in: Ann Intern Med. 2011 Sep 20;**155**(6):408

[5] Inker LA, Schmid CH, Tighiouart H, Eckfeldt JH, Feldman HI, Greene T, et al. Estimating glomerular filtration rate from serum creatinine and cystatin C. New England Journal of Medicine. 2012;**367**(1):20-29

[6] Inker LA, Eneanya ND, Coresh J, Tighiouart H, Wang D, Sang Y, et al. New creatinine- and cystatin C–based equations to estimate GFR without race. New England Journal of Medicine. 2021;**385**(19):1737-1749

[7] Pottel H, Björk J, Rule AD, Ebert N, Eriksen BO, Dubourg L, et al. Cystatin C–based equation to estimate GFR without the inclusion of race and sex. New England Journal of Medicine. 2023;**388**(4):333-343

[8] Mujaj B, Yang WY, Zhang ZY, Wei FF, Thijs L, Verhamme P, et al. Renal function in relation to low-level environmental lead exposure. Nephrology, Dialysis, Transplantation : Official Publication of the European Dialysis and Transplant Association—European Renal Association. 2019;**34**(6):941-946

[9] Pinto-Sietsma SJ, Navis G, Janssen WM, de Zeeuw D, Gans RO, de Jong PE. A central body fat distribution is related to renal function impairment, even in lean subjects. American Journal of Kidney Diseases : The Official Journal of the National Kidney Foundation. 2003;**41**(4):733-741

[10] Mueller-Peltzer K, von Krüchten R, Lorbeer R, Rospleszcz S, Schulz H, Peters A, et al. Adipose tissue is associated with kidney function parameters. Scientific Reports. 2023;**13**(1):9151

[11] Fox CS, Massaro JM, Hoffmann U, Pou KM, Maurovich-Horvat P, Liu CY, et al. Abdominal visceral and subcutaneous adipose tissue compartments: Association with metabolic risk factors in the Framingham heart study. Circulation. 2007;**116**(1):39-48

[12] Iglesias P, Díez JJ. Adipose tissue in renal disease: Clinical significance and prognostic implications. Nephrology Dialysis Transplantation. 2010;**25**(7):2066-2077

[13] Kushner RF, Roth JL. Assessment of the obese patient. Endocrinology and Metabolism Clinics of North America. 2003;**32**(4):915-933

[14] Pavenstädt H. Roles of the podocyte in glomerular function. American Journal of Physiology-Renal Physiology. 2000;**278**(2):F173-F1F9

[15] Kriz W, Lehir M. Pathways to nephron loss starting from glomerular diseases—Insights from animal models. Kidney International. 2005;**67**(2):404-419

[16] Kreiner FF, Schytz PA, Heerspink HJL, von Scholten BJ, Idorn T. Obesity-related kidney disease: Current understanding and future perspectives. Biomedicine. 2023;**11**(9):2498

[17] Lambers Heerspink HJ, Gansevoort RT. Albuminuria is an appropriate therapeutic target in patients with CKD: The pro view. Clinical Journal of the American Society of Nephrology. 2015;**10**(6):1079-1088

[18] Wei L, Li Y, Yu Y, Xu M, Chen H, Li L, et al. Obesity-related Glomerulopathy: From mechanism to therapeutic target. Diabetes, Metabolic Syndrome and Obesity. 28 Oct 2021;**14**:4371-4380. DOI: 10.2147/DMSO.S334199

[19] de Vries AP, Ruggenenti P, Ruan XZ, Praga M, Cruzado JM, Bajema IM, et al. Fatty kidney: Emerging role of ectopic lipid in obesity-related renal disease. The Lancet Diabetes & Endocrinology. 2014;**2**(5):417-426

[20] Vinge E, Lindergård B, Nilsson-Ehle P, Grubb A. Relationships among serum cystatin C, serum creatinine, lean tissue mass and glomerular filtration rate in healthy adults. Scandinavian Journal of Clinical and Laboratory Investigation. 1999;**59**(8):587-592

[21] Young JA, Hwang SJ, Sarnak MJ, Hoffmann U, Massaro JM, Levy D, et al. Association of visceral and subcutaneous adiposity with kidney function. Clinical Journal of the American Society of Nephrology: CJASN. 2008;**3**(6):1786-1791

[22] Schmid C, Ghirlanda C, Zwimpfer C, Tschopp O, Zuellig RA, Niessen M. Cystatin C in adipose tissue and stimulation of its production by growth hormone and triiodothyronine in 3T3-L1 cells. Molecular and Cellular Endocrinology. 2019;**482**:28-36

[23] Bays H, Ballantyne C. Adiposopathy: Why do adiposity and obesity cause metabolic disease? Future Lipidology. 2006;**1**(4):389-420

[24] Calle C, Carranza MC, Simón MA, Torres A, Mayor P. Decreased insulin binding and antilipolytic response in adipocytes from patients with Cushing's syndrome. Bioscience Reports. 1987;**7**(9):713-719

[25] Rebuffé-Scrive M, Krotkiewski M, Elfverson J, Björntorp P. Muscle and adipose tissue morphology and metabolism in Cushing's syndrome. The Journal of Clinical Endocrinology and Metabolism. 1988;**67**(6):1122-1128

[26] Lebovitz HE, Banerji MA. Point: Visceral adiposity is causally related to insulin resistance. Diabetes Care. 2005;**28**(9):2322-2325

[27] Smas CM, Sul HS. Control of adipocyte differentiation. The Biochemical Journal. 1995;**309**(Pt 3):697-710

[28] Engeli S, Schling P, Gorzelniak K, Boschmann M, Janke J, Ailhaud G, et al. The adipose-tissue renin-angiotensin-aldosterone system: Role in the metabolic syndrome? The International Journal of Biochemistry & Cell Biology. 2003;**35**(6):807-825

[29] Kershaw EE, Flier JS. Adipose tissue as an endocrine organ. The Journal of Clinical Endocrinology and Metabolism. 2004;**89**(6):2548-2556

[30] Engeli S. Role of the renin-angiotensin-aldosterone system in the metabolic syndrome. Contributions to Nephrology. 2006;**151**:122-134

[31] Strazzullo P, Galletti F. Impact of the renin-angiotensin system on lipid and carbohydrate metabolism. Current Opinion in Nephrology and Hypertension. 2004;**13**(3):325-332

[32] von Krüchten R, Lorbeer R, Müller-Peltzer K, Rospleszcz S, Storz C, Askani E, et al. Association between adipose tissue depots and dyslipidemia: The KORA-MRI population-based study. Nutrients. 2022;**14**(4):797

[33] Coatmellec-Taglioni G, Ribière C. Factors that influence the risk of hypertension in obese individuals. Current Opinion in Nephrology and Hypertension. 2003;**12**(3):305-308

[34] Mende CW, Einhorn D. Fatty kidney disease: A new renal and endocrine clinical entity? Describing the role of the kidney in obesity, metabolic syndrome, and type 2 diabetes. Endocrine Practice: Official Journal of the American College of Endocrinology and the American Association of Clinical Endocrinologists. 2019;**25**(8):854-858

[35] Foster MC, Hwang S-J, Porter SA, Massaro JM, Hoffmann U, Fox CS. Fatty kidney, hypertension, and chronic kidney disease. Hypertension. 2011;**58**(5):784-790

[36] Foster MC, Hwang SJ, Porter SA, Massaro JM, Hoffmann U, Fox CS. Fatty kidney, hypertension, and chronic kidney disease: The Framingham heart study. Hypertension. 2011;**58**(5):784-790

[37] Scheja L, Heeren J. The endocrine function of adipose tissues in health and cardiometabolic disease. Nature Reviews Endocrinology. 2019;**15**(9):507-524

[38] Chait A, den Hartigh LJ. Adipose tissue distribution, inflammation and its metabolic consequences, including diabetes and cardiovascular disease. Frontiers in Cardiovascular Medicine. 25 Feb 2020;7:22. DOI: 10.3389/fcvm.2020.00022

[39] Przybyciński J, Dziedziejko V, Puchałowicz K, Domański L. Adiponectin in chronic kidney disease. International Journal of Molecular Sciences. 9 Dec 2020;**21**(24):9375. DOI: 10.3390/ijms21249375

[40] Rutkowski JM, Wang ZV, Park ASD, Zhang J, Zhang D, Hu MC, et al. Adiponectin promotes functional recovery after Podocyte ablation. Journal of the American Society of Nephrology. 2013;**24**(2):268-282

[41] Obradovic M, Sudar-Milovanovic E, Soskic S, Essack M, Arya S, Stewart AJ, et al. Leptin and obesity: Role and clinical implication. Frontiers in Endocrinology (Lausanne). 18 May 2021;**12**:585887. DOI: 10.3389/fendo.2021.585887

[42] Pan WW, Myers MG Jr. Leptin and the maintenance of elevated body weight. Nature Reviews Neuroscience. 2018;**19**(2):95-105

[43] Bell BB, Rahmouni K. Leptin as a mediator of obesity-induced hypertension. Current Obesity Reports. 2016;**5**(4):397-404

[44] Kiernan K, MacIver NJ. The role of the Adipokine leptin in immune cell function in health and disease. Frontiers in Immunology. 29 Jan 2021;**11**:622468. DOI: 10.3389/fimmu.2020.622468

[45] Abella V, Scotece M, Conde J, Pino J, Gonzalez-Gay MA, Gómez-Reino JJ, et al. Leptin in the interplay of inflammation, metabolism and immune system disorders. Nature Reviews Rheumatology. 2017;**13**(2):100-109

[46] Cantero-Navarro E, Rayego-Mateos S, Orejudo M, Tejedor-Santamaria L, Tejera-Muñoz A, Sanz AB, et al. Role of macrophages and related cytokines in kidney disease. Frontiers in Medicine. 8 Jul 2021;**8**:688060. DOI: 10.3389/fmed.2021.688060

[47] Furman D, Campisi J, Verdin E, Carrera-Bastos P, Targ S, Franceschi C, et al. Chronic inflammation in the etiology of disease across the life span. Nature Medicine. 2019;**25**(12):1822-1832

[48] Fain JN, Bahouth SW, Madan AK. TNFalpha release by the nonfat cells of human adipose tissue. International Journal of obesity and related metabolic disorders: Journal of the International Association for the Study of Obesity. 2004;**28**(4):616-622

[49] Fain JN, Tichansky DS, Madan AK. Most of the interleukin 1 receptor antagonist, cathepsin S, macrophage migration inhibitory factor, nerve growth factor, and interleukin 18 release by explants of human adipose tissue is by the non–fat cells, not by the adipocytes. Metabolism. 2006;**55**(8):1113-1121

[50] Festa A, D'Agostino R Jr, Tracy RP, Haffner SM. Elevated levels of acute-phase proteins and plasminogen activator inhibitor-1 predict the development of type 2 diabetes: The insulin resistance atherosclerosis study. Diabetes. 2002;**51**(4):1131-1137

[51] Forouhi NG, Sattar N, McKeigue PM. Relation of C-reactive protein to body fat distribution and features of the metabolic syndrome in Europeans and south Asians. International Journal of Obesity and Related Metabolic Disorders: Journal of the International Association for the Study of Obesity. 2001;**25**(9):1327-1331

[52] Matsuzawa Y. Adipocytokines: Emerging therapeutic targets. Current Atherosclerosis Reports. 2005;**7**(1):58-62

[53] Bays H, Blonde L, Rosenson R. Adiposopathy: How do diet, exercise and weight loss drug therapies improve metabolic disease in overweight patients? Expert Review of Cardiovascular Therapy. 2006;**4**(6):871-895

[54] Hall JE, do Carmo JM, da Silva AA, Wang Z, Hall ME. Obesity-induced hypertension: Interaction of neurohumoral and renal mechanisms. Circulation Research. 2015;**116**(6):991-1006

[55] Giacchetti G, Faloia E, Mariniello B, Sardu C, Gatti C, Camilloni MA, et al. Overexpression of the renin-angiotensin system in human visceral adipose tissue in normal and overweight subjects. American Journal of Hypertension. 2002;**15**(5):381-388

[56] Hall JE, do Carmo JM, da Silva AA, Wang Z, Hall ME. Obesity, kidney dysfunction and hypertension: Mechanistic links. Nature Reviews Nephrology. 2019;**15**(6):367-385

[57] Sharma M, Singh V, Sharma R, Koul A, McCarthy ET, Savin VJ, et al. Glomerular biomechanical stress and lipid mediators during cellular changes leading to chronic kidney disease. Biomedicine. 9 Feb 2022;**10**(2):407. DOI: 10.3390/biomedicines10020407

[58] Kahn SE, Hull RL, Utzschneider KM. Mechanisms linking obesity to insulin resistance and type 2 diabetes. Nature. 2006;**444**(7121):840-846

[59] Lay AC, Coward RJM. The evolving importance of insulin signaling in Podocyte health and disease. Frontiers in Endocrinology (Lausanne). 21 Nov 2018;**9**:693. DOI: 10.3389/fendo.2018.00693

[60] Piwkowska A, Rogacka D, Kasztan M, Angielski S, Jankowski M. Insulin increases glomerular filtration barrier permeability through dimerization of protein kinase G type Iα subunits. Biochimica et Biophysica Acta (BBA) - Molecular Basis of Disease. 2013;**1832**(6):791-804

[61] Rogacka D. Insulin resistance in glomerular podocytes: Potential mechanisms of induction. Archives of Biochemistry and Biophysics. 2021;**710**:109005

[62] Morrisey K, Evans RA, Wakefield L, Phillips AO. Translational regulation of renal proximal tubular epithelial cell transforming growth factor-beta1 generation by insulin. The American Journal of Pathology. 2001;**159**(5):1905-1915

[63] Meuwese CL, Carrero JJ. Chronic kidney disease and hypothalamic–pituitary Axis dysfunction: The chicken or the egg? Archives of Medical Research. 2013;**44**(8):591-600

[64] Schultheiss UT, Steinbrenner I, Nauck M, Schneider MP, Kotsis F, Baid-Agrawal S, et al. Thyroid function, renal events and mortality in chronic kidney disease patients: The German chronic kidney disease study. Clinical Kidney Journal. 2020;**14**(3):959-968

[65] Lo JC, Chertow GM, Go AS, Hsu C-Y. Increased prevalence of subclinical and clinical hypothyroidism in persons with chronic kidney disease. Kidney International. 2005;**67**(3):1047-1052

[66] Santini F, Marzullo P, Rotondi M, Ceccarini G, Pagano L, Ippolito S, et al. Mechanisms in endocrinology: The crosstalk between thyroid gland and adipose tissue: Signal integration in health and disease. European Journal of Endocrinology. 2014;**171**(4):R137-RR52

[67] Schultheiss UT, Daya N, Grams ME, Seufert J, Steffes M, Coresh J, et al. Thyroid function, reduced kidney function and incident chronic kidney disease in a community-based population: The atherosclerosis risk in communities study. Nephrology Dialysis Transplantation. 2016;**32**(11):1874-1881

[68] Fricker M, Wiesli P, Brändle M, Schwegler B, Schmid C. Impact of thyroid dysfunction on serum cystatin C. Kidney International. 2003;**63**(5):1944-1947

[69] Liu S, Shen S, Yan Y, Sun C, Lu Z, Feng H, et al. Triiodothyronine (T3) promotes brown fat hyperplasia via thyroid hormone receptor-mediated adipocyte progenitor cell proliferation. Nature Communications. 2022;**13**(1):3394

Chapter 7

Resistin in Early Diabetic Chronic Kidney Disease: Exploring the Link with Nutritional Status and Cardiovascular Outcome

Roberto Calças Marques, Henriques Borges, Rita Afonso, José Soares, Eduarda Carias, Hermínio Carrasqueira and Ana Paula Silva

Abstract

High resistin levels have been associated with malnutrition, inflammation, and cardiovascular risk in patients with chronic kidney disease (CKD). This study aimed to elucidate the relationship between serum resistin levels and the Patient-Generated Subjective Global Assessment (PG-SGA), a validated nutritional assessment tool in this population. It also investigates the role of resistin as a potential predictor of cardiovascular mortality in early-stage diabetic CKD. Prospective observational study that included 217 type 2 diabetic patients with mild to moderate CKD. Patients were divided into three groups according to PG-SGA: well-nourished (category A), moderately malnourished or suspected of being malnourished (category B), or severely malnourished (category C). The severely malnourished group had higher resistin levels, and resistin was positively correlated with IL-6, PG-SGA score, left ventricular mass index, and pulse pressure, while negatively correlating with vitamin D and estimated glomerular filtration rate (eGFR). We found that high resistin levels (HR = 1.350; 95% CI 1.187–1.535), PG-SGA greater than 10 (HR = 4.858; 95% CI 1.664–14.185), and higher HOMA-IR (HR = 1.099; 95% CI 1.007–4.001) were significant independent predictors of cardiovascular mortality. The study suggests that high resistin levels are associated with malnutrition in mild to moderate CKD and independently predict cardiovascular mortality in this population.

Keywords: resistin, chronic fidney disease, type 2 diabetes, nutritional status, cardiovascular outcome

1. Introduction

Cardiovascular disease is the leading cause of death in chronic kidney disease (CKD) [1]. Alongside the classic cardiovascular risk factors, such as hypertension, dyslipidemia, diabetes, and insulin resistance, inflammation and malnutrition, are recognized factors associated with increased morbidity and mortality in these patients [2, 3].

Resistin, an adipokine discovered two decades ago, is characterized as a 12.5 kilodalton cysteine-rich protein, which has been notably implicated in insulin resistance, particularly in murine models [4]. Nevertheless, human data presents a divergence of findings concerning its association with insulin resistance and obesity [5]. Paradoxically, resistin emerges as a pivotal participant in the immune system, being acknowledged as a pro-inflammatory adipokine [6]. While its principal source of secretion is adipocytes, it is noteworthy that monocytes, macrophages, bone marrow cells, and cardiomyocytes can also contribute to its secretion [7–9].

Among individuals with CKD, resistin demonstrates a correlation with inflammation as numerous studies elucidate an association between its serum levels and serum tumor necrosis factor-alpha and interleukin 6 (IL-6) levels [10, 11]. Elevated levels of resistin have also been linked to malnutrition in dialysis patients [12, 13]. Among elderly nondiabetic CKD patients, elevated circulating levels of resistin appear to be an independent predictor of cardiovascular and all-cause mortality [14]. Furthermore, resistin exhibits a robust association with mortality and graft loss in kidney transplant recipients [15].

The kidney disease outcomes and quality initiative (KDOQI) recommends the subjective global assessment (SGA) instrument as the gold standard for nutritional assessment in CKD, a tool that is now available as the web-based program Scored Patient-Generated Subjective Global Assessment (PG-SGA), which has already been validated in this population [16–18].

This study aims to elucidate the relationship between serum resistin levels and malnutrition, explore its association with inflammation, and evaluate the potential of resistin as a prognostic factor for cardiovascular mortality in early diabetic CKD.

2. Materials and methods

2.1 Study population

In this observational prospective study, we included patients with type 2 diabetes who were recruited between January 2015 and June 2022 with a diagnosis of mild to moderate CKD (stages 2–3) in a stable clinical condition followed in our outpatient clinic.

The exclusion criteria were as follows: age 75 years, estimated glomerular filtration rate (eGFR) ≤ 29 or > 90 mL/min, type 1 diabetes, nondiabetic renal disease, and known neoplastic, infectious, or chronic inflammatory diseases.

The study procedure encompassed data collection and patient interviews to evaluate nutritional status through the utilization of the PG-SGA. This tool includes objective and subjective information. The first section focuses on patient grading and comprises data concerning the patient's medical history, covering factors such as weight variations, changes in dietary habits, gastrointestinal symptoms, physical activities, and functional capacity. The second section, based on physician grading, encompasses information related to the patient's disease status such as comorbidities and advanced age, metabolic demands, as well as findings from a physical examination, including observations of subcutaneous fat loss and indications of muscle wasting. Patients were then categorized into well-nourished (category A), moderately malnourished or suspected of being malnourished (category B), or severely malnourished (category C). The PG-SGA score ranges from 0 to 36, with a higher score indicating more severe malnutrition.

Serum samples were collected from fasting patients. Plasma resistin levels were determined by enzyme-linked immunosorbent assay. GFR was estimated using the National Kidney Foundation recommended Chronic Kidney Disease Epidemiology Collaboration (CKD-EPI) equation [19].

Approval was obtained from the local ethics committee. All principles of the declaration of Helsinki of 1975 were followed and study procedures were only conducted after obtaining patients' written informed consent.

2.2 Statistical analysis

Categorical variables are expressed as frequencies and percentages, while continuous variables are presented as mean and standard deviation (SD) or median and interquartile range (IQR).

We used one-way analysis (ANOVA) and post hoc analysis with the Scheffe test to compare the groups. Pearson's correlation test was performed to measure the association between the identified variables and resistin levels.

Univariate and multivariate Cox regression analyses were performed to determine the association between serum resistin levels and cardiovascular mortality.

Statistical analysis was performed using 'Statistical Package for the Social Science' version 29.0 for Windows (SPSS, Chicago, IL, USA). A P-value less than 0.05 was considered statistically significant.

3. Results

Two hundred and seventeen (217) patients with type 2 diabetes and CKD stage 2–3 were included in the study after confirming they did not meet any of the exclusion criteria.

The mean age was 56.01 ± 24.05 years, of whom 60.4% (131) were male. 36.9% (n = 80) of patients had hypertension and the mean follow-up was 54.30 ± 24.05 months.

Table 1 shows patients' demographic and clinical parameters, and a comparison between groups. 36.9% (n = 80) of patients had hypertension.

A total of 43 (19.8%) patients died during the course of the study.

The severely malnourished group had lower eGFR (29.16 vs. 48.48 mL/min/1.73m^2, $p < 0.001$); higher levels of resistin (6.25 vs. 4.49 ng/mL, $p = 0.004$), parathormone (176.22 vs. 115.23 pg./mL, $p < 0.001$), phosphorus (4.47 vs. 3.91 mg/dL, $p = 0.001$), HOMA-IR (2.46 vs. 1.52, $p = 0.009$) and IL-6 (7.23 vs. 4.56 pg./ml, $p < 0.001$); lower levels of hemoglobin (11.94 vs. 12.97 g/dL, $p < 0.001$), calcium (8.58 vs. 9.05 mg/dl, $p = 0.026$) and 25(OH)D3 (18.46 vs. 21.52 ng/mL, $p = 0.035$); higher left ventricular hypertrophy (LVMI 115.19 vs. 95.59 g/m^2, $p < 0.001$) and higher pulse pressure (71.60 vs. 56.58, $p = 0.005$) when compared to the well-nourished group. No statistical differences were observed between sexes.

Pearson's correlation analysis revealed significant associations between resistin and various biochemical and clinical parameters. A moderate positive correlation was observed between resistin and IL-6 ($r = 0.591$, $p < 0.001$), as well as between resistin and LVMI ($r = 0.489$, $p < 0.001$). Additionally, weaker positive correlations were identified between resistin and both pulse pressure ($r = 0.310$, $p < 0.001$) and

	Category A (well-nourished) N = 71 (32.7%)	Category B (moderately nourished) N = 58 (26.7%)	Category C (malnourished) N = 88 (40.6%)	ANOVA p-value	Category A vs. -C p-value
Age, years	49.08 ± 26.34	54.30 ± 18.83	60.92 ± 20.61	< 0.001	< 0.001
eGFR, mL/min/1.73m^2	48.48 ± 23.93	40.06 ± 22.60	29.16 ± 15.34	< 0.001	< 0.001
PG-SGA score, median	3	9	11	< 0.001	< 0.001
Resistin, ng/mL	4.49 ± 3.18	5.63 ± 3.38	6.25 ± 3.47	0.004	0.004
IL-6, pg./mL	4.56 ± 3.33	6.65 ± 3.21	7.23 ± 3.32	< 0.001	< 0.001
HOMA-IR	1.52 ± 1.53	2.19 ± 1.70	2.46 ± 1.90	0.008	0.009
Hemoglobin, g/dL	12.97 ± 1.61	12.30 ± 1.51	11.94 ± 1.60	< 0.001	< 0.001
Ferritin, ng/mL	194.80 ± 134.37	169.65 ± 167.76	189.36 ± 162.42	0.544	0.992
LVMI, g/m^2	95.59 ± 24.54	108.82 ± 27.66	115.19 ± 23.27	< 0.001	< 0.001
Pulse pressure, mmHg	56.58 ± 21.37	60.99 ± 18.63	71.60 ± 17.51	< 0.001	< 0.001
Total cholesterol, mg/dL	163.04 ± 70.78	148.07 ± 74.21	115.29 ± 80.61	< 0.001	< 0.001
Calcium, mg/dL	9.05 ± 1.11	8.92 ± 1.06	8.58 ± 1.14	0.020	0.026
Phosphorus, mg/dL	3.91 ± 0.74	4.17 ± 0.82	4.47 ± 1.18	0.001	0.001
25(OH)D3, ng/mL	21.52 ± 6.38	20.85 ± 7.13	18.46 ± 8.40	0.024	0.035
PTH, ng/mL	115.23 ± 88.21	135.36 ± 70.73	176.22 ± 89.54	< 0.001	< 0.001

Values are means ± SD unless specified otherwise. eGFR: estimated glomerular filtration rate HOMA-IR: homeostatic model assessment for insulin resistance; IL-6: interleukin-6; LVMI: left ventricular mass index; PG-SGA: Patient-Generated Subjective Global Assessment; PTH: parathyroid hormone.

Table 1.
Patients' demographic and clinical characteristics of each cohort.

	HR (CI 95%)	P-value
Resistin levels	1.350 (1.187–1.535)	< 0.001
PG-SGA score		
0–10 points	Ref.	
> 10 points	4.858 (1.664–14.185)	0.004
HOMA-IR	1.099 (1.007–4.001)	0.002

Adjusted to age, eGFR and IL-6. HOMA-IR: homeostatic model assessment for insulin resistance; HR: hazard ratio; IL-6: interleukin-6; PG-SGA: Patient-Generated Subjective Global Assessment.

Table 2.
Independent predictors of cardiovascular mortality by multivariate cox regression in early CKD.

PG-SGA score ($r = 0.217$, $p < 0.001$). Conversely, a strong negative correlation was observed between resistin and vitamin D ($r = -0.854$, $p < 0.001$), and a weaker negative correlation was found between resistin and eGFR ($r = -0.246$, $p < 0.001$). No association was found between resistin and HOMA-IR and total cholesterol.

On multivariable modeling, we found that higher resistin levels (HR = 1.350; 95% CI 1.187–1.535), PG-SGA score greater than 10 (HR = 4.858; 95% CI 1.664–14.185), and higher HOMA-IR (HR = 1.099; 95% CI 1.007–4.001) were significant independent predictors of cardiovascular mortality when adjusted for age, IL-6 and eGFR (**Table 2**).

4. Discussion

Resistin has gained attention as a potential link between malnutrition, inflammation, and cardiovascular risk in patients with CKD [12, 20, 21].

Increased resistin levels may be involved in the development of malnutrition-inflammation states and, consequently, protein-energy wasting, a condition of paramount significance in the context of managing this population [21, 22]. Our results corroborate this, showing higher plasma resistin levels in the malnourished group and a positive association with both IL-6 and PG-SGA scores. Increased resistin levels were also correlated with left ventricular hypertrophy and pulse pressure, both of which are independent markers of cardiovascular risk in CKD [23, 24].

A strong inverse correlation was identified between resistin and vitamin D levels. Multiple investigations have reported similar findings, thereby bolstering the hypothesis that vitamin D may play a role in modulating resistin [25, 26]. Nevertheless, a study conducted by Vaidya A. et al. documented a positive correlation between these factors, complicating the formulation of their interrelationship [27].

A negative association between resistin and eGFR was also established, consistent with several data suggesting that this relationship represents a physiological mechanism due to the elimination of resistin by the kidneys [28, 29]. Stepien et al. also observed a negative correlation between resistin and eGFR, although this difference did not reach statistical significance [30]. They attributed this nonsignificant result to factors such as the sample size and the early stage of CKD. In fact, the comparison of a group with early-stage CKD to a group without CKD may account for this finding.

Given resistin's known association with inflammation and the well-established link between inflammation and the pathogenesis of atherosclerosis, it has been advocated that resistin could be a useful predictive biomarker of adverse cardiovascular outcome in this population. Our study explored this idea, showing that higher serum resistin levels are independently associated with cardiovascular mortality in early diabetic CKD patients. PG-SGA score greater than 10 was also associated with cardiovascular mortality. Similar result was obtained by Rodrigues et al., who enrolled 146 women with gynecologic cancer and found a significant association between PG-SGA score (> 10 points versus 0–10 points) and all-cause mortality within 1 year [31].

Several limitations of this study need to be acknowledged. Firstly, it was a small-sample observational, prospective study, potentially compromising the strength of some statistical analysis. Secondly, resistin levels were assessed on a single occasion, and confounding factors at the time of collection not taken into account in this study may have influenced our results. Thirdly, it is important to note that this study is prognostic rather than an etiologic study.

5. Conclusion

The study suggests that high resistin levels are associated with malnutrition in mild to moderate CKD and independently predict cardiovascular mortality in this population.

Conflict of interest

The authors declare no conflict of interest.

Author details

Roberto Calças Marques[1*], Henriques Borges[1], Rita Afonso[1], José Soares[1], Eduarda Carias[2], Hermínio Carrasqueira[1] and Ana Paula Silva[1,3]

1 Nephrology Deparment, Centro Hospitalar Universitário do Algarve, Faro, Portugal

2 Nephrology Deparment, Centro Hospitalar do Tâmega e Sousa, Penafiel, Portugal

3 Deparment of Biomedical Sciences and Medicine, Universidade do Algarve, Faro, Portugal

*Address all correspondence to: rcmarques@chua.min-saude.pt

References

[1] Jankowski J, Floege J, Fliser D, et al. Cardiovascular disease in chronic kidney disease: Pathophysiological insights and therapeutic options. Circulation. 2021;**143**:1157-1172. DOI: 10.1161/circulationaha.120.050686

[2] Kalantar-Zadeh K, Kopple JD, Block G, Humphreys MH. A malnutrition-inflammation score is correlated with morbidity and mortality in maintenance hemodialysis patients. American Journal of Kidney Diseases. 2001;**38**:1251-1263. DOI: 10.1053/ajkd.2001.29222

[3] Jagadeswaran D, Indhumathi E, Hemamalini AJ, et al. Inflammation and nutritional status assessment by malnutrition inflammation score and its outcome in pre-dialysis chronic kidney disease patients. Clinical Nutrition. 2019;**38**:341-347. DOI: 10.1016/j.clnu.2018.01.001

[4] Steppan CM, Bailey ST, Bhat S, et al. The hormone resistin links obesity to diabetes. Nature. 2001;**409**:307-312. DOI: 10.1038/35053000

[5] Acquarone E, Monacelli F, Borghi R, et al. Resistin: A reappraisal. Mechanisms of Ageing and Development. 2019;**178**:46-63. DOI: 10.1016/j.mad.2019.01.004

[6] Filkova M, Haluzik M, Gay S, Senolt L. The role of resistin as a regulator of inflammation: Implications for various human pathologies. Clinical Immunology. 2009;**133**:157-170. DOI: 10.1016/j.clim.2009.07.013

[7] Patel L, Buckels AC, Kinghorn IJ, et al. Resistin is expressed in human macrophages and directly regulated by PPAR gamma activators. Biochemical and Biophysical Research Communications. 2003;**300**:472-476. DOI: 10.1016/s0006-291x(02)02841-3

[8] Thommesen L, Stunes AK, Monjo M, et al. Expression and regulation of resistin in osteoblasts and osteoclasts indicate a role in bone metabolism. Journal of Cellular Biochemistry. 2006;**99**:824-834. DOI: 10.1002/jcb.20915

[9] Kim M, Oh JK, Sakata S, et al. Role of resistin in cardiac contractility and hypertrophy. Journal of Molecular and Cellular Cardiology. 2008;**45**:270-280. DOI: 10.1016/j.yjmcc.2008.05.006

[10] Schwartz DR, Lazar MA. Human resistin: Found in translation from mouse to man. Trends in Endocrinology and Metabolism. 2011;**22**:259-265. DOI: 10.1016/j.tem.2011.03.005

[11] Fargnoli JL, Sun Q, Olenczuk D, et al. Resistin is associated with biomarkers of inflammation while total and high-molecular weight adiponectin are associated with biomarkers of inflammation, insulin resistance, and endothelial function. European Journal of Endocrinology. 2010;**162**:281-288. DOI: 10.1530/EJE-09-0555

[12] Liakopoulos V, Mertens PR, Eleftheriadis T, et al. Is there a link between inflammation, plasma resistin levels, and protein malnutrition in hemodialysis patients. Kidney International. 2006;**70**:1371-1372. DOI: 10.1038/sj.ki.5001584

[13] Kaynar K, Kural BV, Ulusoy S, et al. Is there any interaction of resistin and adiponectin levels with protein-energy wasting among patients with chronic kidney disease. Hemodialysis

International. 2014;**18**:153-162. DOI: 10.1111/hdi.12072

[14] Marouga A, Dalamaga M, Kastania AN, et al. Circulating resistin is a significant predictor of mortality independently from cardiovascular comorbidities in elderly, non-diabetic subjects with chronic kidney disease. Biomarkers. 2016;**21**:73-79. DOI: 10.3109/1354750X.2015.1118536

[15] Nagy K, Ujszaszi A, Czira MA, et al. Association between serum resistin level and outcomes in kidney transplant recipients. Transplant International. 2016;**29**:352-361. DOI: 10.1111/tri.12728

[16] Ikizler TA, Cuppari L. The 2020 updated KDOQI clinical practice guidelines for nutrition in chronic kidney disease. Blood Purification. 2021;**50**:667-671. DOI: 10.1159/000513698

[17] Rashid I, Tiwari P, D'Cruz S, Jaswal S. Nutritional status, symptom burden, and predictive validity of the PtGlobal web tool/PG-SGA in CKD patients: A hospital based cross sectional study. PLOS Global Public Health. 2023;**3**:e0001301. DOI: 10.1371/journal.pgph.0001301

[18] Desbrow B, Bauer J, Blum C, et al. Assessment of nutritional status in hemodialysis patients using patientgenerated subjective global assessment. Journal of Renal Nutrition. 2005;**15**:211-216. DOI: 10.1053/j.jrn.2004.10.005

[19] Levey AS, Stevens LA, Schmid CH, et al. A new equation to estimate glomerular filtration rate. Annals of Internal Medicine. 2009;**150**:604-612. DOI: 10.7326/0003-4819-150-9-200905050-00006

[20] Park HK, Kwak MK, Kim HJ, Ahima RS. Linking resistin, inflammation, and cardiometabolic diseases. The Korean Journal of Internal Medicine. 2017;**32**:239-247. DOI: 10.3904/kjim.2016.229

[21] Romejko K, Rymarz A, Szamotulska K, et al. Resistin contribution to cardiovascular risk in chronic kidney disease male patients. Cell. 2023;**12**:999. DOI: 10.3390/cells12070999

[22] Kamimura MA, Nerbass FB. Nutritional assessment in chronic kidney disease: The protagonism of longitudinal measurement. Jornal Brasileiro de Nefrologia. 2020;**42**:4-5. DOI: 10.1590/2175-8239-jbn-2020-0010

[23] Fernandez-Fresnedo G, Rodrigo E, De Francisco ALM, et al. Role of pulse pressure on cardiovascular risk in chronic kidney disease patients. Journal of the American Society of Nephrology. 2006;**17**:S246-S249. DOI: 10.1681/ASN.2006080921

[24] Di Lullo L, Gorini A, Russo D, Santoboni A, et al. Left ventricular hypertrophy in chronic kidney disease patients: From pathophysiology to treatment. Cardiorenal Medicine. 2015;**5**:254-266. DOI: 10.1159/000435838

[25] Tariq S, Tariq S, Khaliq S, et al. Association between vitamin D and Resistin in postmenopausal females with altered bone health. Frontiers in Endocrinology (Lausanne). 2020;**11**:615440. DOI: 10.3389/fendo.2020.615440

[26] Ismail MM, Hamid TAA, Ibrahim AA, Marzouk H. Serum adipokines and vitamin D levels in patients with type 1 diabetes mellitus. Archives of Medical Science. 2017;**13**:738-744. DOI: 10.5114/aoms.2016.60680

[27] Vaidya A, Pojoga L, Underwood PC, et al. The association of plasma resistin

with dietary sodium manipulation, the renin-angiotensin-aldosterone system, and 25-hydroxyvitamin D3 in human hypertension. Clinical Endocrinology. 2011;**74**:294-299. DOI: 10.1111/j.1365-2265.2010.03922.x

[28] Fagerberg B, Fagerlund C, Hulthe J. Resistin and GFR. Kidney International. 2006;**70**:1371. DOI: 10.1038/sj.ki.5001583

[29] Axelsson J, Bergsten A, Qureshi AR, et al. Elevated resistin levels in chronic kidney disease are associated with decreased glomerular filtration rate and inflammation, but not with insulin resistance. Kidney International. 2006;**69**:596-604. DOI: 10.1038/sj.ki.5000089

[30] Stepien M, Stepien A, Wlazel RN, et al. Obesity indices and adipokines in non-diabetic obese patients with early stages of chronic kidney disease. Medical Science Monitor. 2013;**19**:1063-1072. DOI: 10.12659/MSM.889390

[31] Rodrigues CS, Lacerda MS, Chaves GV. Patient generated subjective global assessment as a prognosis tool in women with gynecologic cancer. Nutrition. 2015;**31**:1372-1378. DOI: 10.1016/j.nut.2015.06.001

Section 3

Renoprotection and New Therapeutic Options

Chapter 8

Renoprotective Interventions Efficacy in the Late Stages of CKD

Daria Sergeevna Sadovskaya

Abstract

The efficacy of renoprotective interventions in the late stages of chronic kidney disease (CKD) varies significantly from that in the early stages, with approaches in advanced CKD being insufficiently developed and sometimes conflicting. In a small prospective study, we evaluated the effectiveness of intensive follow-up protocol aimed at reducing CKD progression rates, cardiovascular complications, and improving outcomes among 100 patients with CKD3B-5 stages at a single center. This evaluation was compared with the outcomes of standard nephrology care. Positive changes in modifiable parameters resulting from interventions (such as serum albumin, hemoglobin, and standard bicarbonate) or reductions in negative parameters (like serum phosphate, plasma calcium deviation from target range, uric acid, and systolic blood pressure) were independently associated with a comparable reduction in the decrease of glomerular filtration rate (GFR). For the treatment group, the predicted time to reach the need for renal replacement therapy (RRT) from a conditional GFR of 20 ml/min/1.73 m^2 was 5 months longer than in the regular follow-up group. The distribution of average GFR at the start of dialysis suggested a late and possibly premature start in the control group, with less than 60% of cases being planned. In contrast, the treatment group always had a planned start.

Keywords: CKD progression, glomerular filtration rate, renoprotection, RAAS blockade, sodium-glucose transporter inhibitor, neprilysin inhibitor, selective mineralocorticoid receptor antagonist

1. Introduction

In the new millennium, the death rate from chronic kidney disease (CKD) has nearly doubled and its prevalence increased by 30% to more than 700 million worldwide, surpassing those of diabetes mellitus and chronic obstructive pulmonary disease (COPD) [1]. Cardiovascular diseases (CVDs) now account for almost half of deaths in CKD patients [2]. The cardiovascular risk in CKD, especially below an estimated glomerular filtration rate (eGFR) of 45 ml/min/1.73 m^2 or a urine albumin-to-creatinine ratio (ACR) exceeding 300 mg/g, is significantly higher compared to the non-CKD population.

The impact of traditional and nontraditional risk factors for cardiovascular disease (CVD) differs in CKD. Despite the definite position in Kidney Disease

Improving Global Outcomes Chronic Kidney Disease (KDIGO CKD) guidelines (≤120/80 mmHg) [3], the optimal target blood pressure for hypertension remains uncertain, as it is controversial and based on weak evidence [4, 5]. Standardized blood pressure measurements pose challenges in nonresearch settings, and the recommended target is not readily applicable to routine measurements. This situation may expose multimorbid patients to heightened risks of falls and fractures. Furthermore, achieving the suggested blood pressure target might prove challenging for a significant proportion of CKD patients.

Cardiovascular (CV) risks in patients with CKD involve salt and water retention causing sympathetic activation and stimulation of renin-angiotensin-aldosterone system (RAAS). Uremic toxin retention contributes to increased oxidative stress, inflammation, and platelet activation; phosphate accumulation plays a pivotal role in vascular calcification and parathyroid bone disease. In this chapter, we will limit our discussion to novel mechanisms and approaches related to CKD progression because others were reviewed in detail in the update of KDIGO CKD guidelines. We'll particularly emphasize the advanced stages, aligning with our study's dedication to exploring nephroprotection possibilities on CKD3B-5 stages.

2. Lifestyle modification forms the foundation of nephroprotection

Understanding the impact of exercise in advanced stages of CKD on disease progression remains unclear. A meta-analysis of 18 randomized controlled trials (RCTs) showed insignificant effects on mortality and eGFR. However, physical exercise did enhance peak/maximum oxygen consumption, physical performance, and walking ability in predialysis CKD patients. These improvements could potentially reduce the risk of falls, fractures, and enhance long-term prognosis. An umbrella review of 31 meta-analyses with 120 different outcomes [6] revealed small effect sizes for most cardiorenal outcomes, with generally low-quality studies.

Obesity is an important risk factor for CKD development and progression, only partially explained by the diabetes mellitus and hypertension in obese patients. The adipose tissue also possesses high endocrine functions that contribute to low-grade inflammation with risk of kidney damage. Moreover, the effect of bariatric surgery on elimination of hyperfiltration highly depends on the downregulation of inflammasome signaling [7].

Several randomized controlled trials (RCTs) on sodium-glucose cotransporter 2 (SGL2) inhibitors, glucagon-like peptide-1 (GLP-1) analogues, and bariatric surgery in diabetic kidney disease showed renoprotective effects. The sodium-glucose cotransporter 2 inhibitors (SGLT2i) provided better renal outcomes, while glucagon-like peptide-1 receptor agonists (GLP1-RA) demonstrated better weight loss effect; there is dearth of RCT data concerning combination of SGLT2i plus GLP1-RA (as well as plus bariatric surgery) but the available data are already very promising [8]. Unfortunately, the advanced stage CKD patients are minority in mentioned trials (besides the last SGLT2i trials).

The concept of slowing down the progression of CKD through a low-protein diet has been around since the last century. However, large-scale studies like Modification of Diet in Renal Disease (MDRD) have yielded negative results, and achieving the target protein intake remains challenging.

Limiting protein intake poses the risks of protein-energy wasting. Conversely, patients often restrict protein intake as azotemia worsens. Modern approaches echo those of the past, with consistent goals: a protein intake of 0.6 and 0.3 g /kg/day (the latter, in combination with ketoanalogues of amino acids, to reach equivalent of 0.6 g/kg/day). Monitoring protein intake through daily urea excretion is essential. However, the real-world effectiveness of low-protein diets remains inconclusive. KDIGO CKD guidelines (2024) suggest maintaining a protein intake of 0.8 g/kg/day in adults with CKD G3-G5 stages. Additionally, it's advised not to restrict protein intake in adults with sarcopenia, cachexia, or conditions leading to undernutrition.

Despite lacking hard clinical evidence, there's some indication of the positive impact of plant-based proteins on CKD progression, blood pressure, and acidosis. This insight is highlighted in a review prepared for KDIGO CKD guidelines in 2024 [3], encouraging further research.

Notably, very low-protein diets seem to decrease the number of patients in CKD4–5 stages and the need for renal replacement therapy (RRT). Diets with low-protein content have a modest effect on this indicator, and those with low or very low-protein content do not influence mortality. However, they carry the risk of developing protein-energy wasting.

Reducing sodium intake is crucial in the general population, but in CKD, there is a J-shaped link between adverse outcomes and natremia. Hyponatremia's association with comorbidities like cardiovascular issues and protein-energy wasting may explain this. Salt restriction leads to a decrease in blood pressure, extracellular fluid volume, and albuminuria, with less convincing evidence for slowing CKD progression; the studies conducted on this topic were of relatively short duration. In the studies involving RAAS blockade, salt restriction was beneficial, enhancing the nephrocardioprotective effect. However, a short-term decrease in GFR can be expected due to the elimination of hyperfiltration. Accumulation of sodium in nonionic form within the intradermal layer can act as an internal source explaining delayed manifestation of positive effects after the introduction of dietary restriction [9].

In the general population, the interaction of sodium and potassium influences hypertension development more than sodium levels alone. In CKD, higher potassium intake slows down progression. A diet rich in vegetables and fruits slows down the CKD progression and adds a hypotensive effect to medications. Questions persist about what is positive in a vegetarian diet: potassium-rich food, dietary fiber content (with an effect on the microbiota, inflammation, and intestinal uremic toxins' generation), or a limitation of rapidly absorbed phosphates [10]. Potassium intake reduction becomes relevant in CKD stage 3B, set at 2.5 g/day with kalemia monitoring.

Phosphate consumption, especially from processed products, exceeds needs in the general population, but in CKD, hyperphosphatemia poses greater risks. It accelerates the progression of CKD and counteracts the nephroprotective effect of RAAS blockade. The challenge arises from the need to combat hyperphosphatemia without imposing substantial restrictions on protein intake. Additional dietary control measures involve the use of medications such as phosphate binders and absorption blockers, along with addressing hyperparathyroidism.

Vascular calcification risks in predialysis CKD stages limit the use of calcium-free phosphate binders. Invasive techniques [11] may become relevant for predialysis CKD stages due to restrictions in calcimimetics (due to the outpacing growth of phosphate in comparison with the rate of suppression of hyperparathyroidism) and vitamin D use (due to the risk of hypercalcemia).

The use of synbiotics in CKD stages 3B-4 resulted in a significant transformation of the intestinal microbiome, enriching it with bifidobacteria, lactobacilli, and

Subdoligranulum. This intervention also led to a reduction in the level of indoxyl sulfate in the blood, an improvement in eGFR, and the decrease in C-reactive protein (CRP) levels. The initial studies on this subject, when combined in a meta-analysis, demonstrated positive effects [12]. Additionally, the inclusion of polyunsaturated fatty acids (PUFAs) as supplements in CKD showcased enhancements in lipid profiles and a reduction in oxidative stress [13].

The consumption of easily digestible carbohydrates in the broader population is linked to the development of metabolic syndrome, hypertension, albuminuria, and the onset of CKD. Although there are no direct studies focused on CKD, it's crucial to note that an elevated content of glycation end products in food heightens the risk of death in CKD. Reducing the intake of these compounds in the diet has been shown to improve kidney function and lower inflammatory markers [14]. It's noteworthy that among 120,000 patients with obesity and hypertension, the use of prescribed RAAS blockers increased the risks of developing or progressing CKD [15].

Tobacco smoking is one of the leading causes of preventable deaths, including cardiovascular diseases and cancer. It is associated with proteinuria and a decrease in GFR in the general population and accelerates the progression of established CKD and exacerbates proteinuria. Moreover, smoking reduces the survival rate of kidney transplant recipients and worsens the graft survival. These effects depend on the dose and time and can be attenuated by quitting smoking. Quitting smoking slows down the progression of kidney disease [16].

3. RAAS blockade

As per a meta-analysis network [17], the use of ACE inhibitors (ACEis) or angiotensin II receptor blockers (ARBs) in CKD patients is associated with a decreased risk of kidney failure and cardiovascular events. ACEi, in particular, demonstrated a 28% reduction in the risk for all-cause mortality by 28% and proved to be superior to ARBs across various outcomes. This suggests that ACE inhibitors could be considered the preferred choice for treatment, especially in populations primarily dealing with CKD stages 1-3A. Of note, only quarter of 119 studies included patients with CKD3 or higher. Both ACE inhibitors and ARBs significantly lowered the odds of kidney failure by 39 and 30%, respectively, compared to a placebo. When compared with other active controls, other active controls showed no significant impact on kidney failure. Moreover, both ACE inhibitors and ARBs demonstrated a reduction in major cardiovascular events. While controls did not exhibit a notable effect on the risk of cardiovascular death. In comparisons between ARBs and ACEis, the latter consistently showed higher probabilities of reducing kidney failure, cardiovascular death, or all-cause death. It's crucial to consider potential risks associated with these drugs. Implementing protocols for the prevention and treatment of hyperkalemia can help balance potassium levels and facilitate the initiation or continuation of RAAS blockade in CKD3–5.

A large (involving more than 5000 patients) study of real-world practice [18] showed that the initiation of therapy of RAAS blockers, in comparison with calcium blockers, reduces the risk of dialysis by 21% in progressive CKD3–5, with comparable cardioprotective efficacy. On the contrary, the termination of the RAAS blockade was associated with higher absolute risks of death and serious cardiovascular events, simultaneously, a lower absolute risk of the need for RRT [19]. The negative impact of RAAS blockade on kidney function may only be a matter of necessary dose adjustment, raising questions about the threshold at which the previously effective nephroprotective approach becomes ineffective.

The extent to which intensive blood pressure control, with target levels below 120/80 mmHg, is beneficial or acceptable remains unclear. Attempts to intensify antihypertensive therapy to achieve this goal led to an accelerated decrease in kidney function (while reducing the risks of cardiovascular events) and an increase in episodes of acute kidney injury (AKI). The nephroprotective effect of antihypertensive therapy is lower with proteinuria of less than 1 g/day. The discussion on this topic was sharpened by the release of KDIGO clinical recommendations on blood pressure in CKD [20], which emphasized the importance of standardized measurement and strict control of blood pressure. However, the target systolic blood pressure level of less than 120 mmHg is controversial. The recommendation is based on weak evidence and may not be applicable to most patients with CKD. Striving for such a target in routine practice may expose multimorbid patients to adverse events, including falls and fractures, and is often unattainable for most CKD patients [4].

In 2019, a meta-analysis of randomized controlled trials (RCTs) failed to conclusively support the use of RAAS blockers as nephroprotective therapy in CKD3–4 and even in populations with CKD1–4. The odds ratio (OR) is 1.05; 95% confidence interval (CI) 0.99–1.11. The same meta-analysis confirmed the effectiveness of lipid-lowering therapy (OR 1.04; 95% CI 1.00–1.08) and glycemic control (OR 1.06; 95% CI 1.02–1.10) [21].

A network meta-analysis systematically evaluates the efficacy of various interventions, even in the absence of direct head-to-head comparisons. In a recent publication addressing such comprehensive comparisons [22], it was observed that ACEi and ARBs demonstrate nephrocardioprotection in the broader category of CKD patients. However, uncertainties persist regarding the effectiveness and safety of these drugs specifically in individuals with CKD3–4.

4. Angiotensin receptor/neprilysin inhibitor

For over two decades, therapy with ACE inhibitors (ACEis) and angiotensin II receptor blockers (ARBs) has been employed in patients with chronic heart failure (HF) and reduced ejection fraction to mitigate the risk of mortality. Neurohormonal activation resulting from ACEi or ARB monotherapy contributes to lingering cardiovascular risk, particularly in patients with concomitant resistant hypertension.

In this context, newer agents, such as ARNI (angiotensin receptor/neprilysin inhibitor), may offer additional benefits by counteracting neurohormonal activation stemming from ACEi or ARB monotherapy. These agents operate by enhancing cyclic guanosine monophosphate (cGMP) levels in cardiomyocytes and inhibiting the renin-angiotensin-aldosterone system (RAAS). ARNI, exemplified by the first-in-class combination of sacubitril and valsartan, has demonstrated superiority over ACEi or ARB in reducing inflammation and cardiorenal fibrosis in animal studies.

Due to the additional benefits of ARNI, it may potentially achieve a more significant reduction in blood pressure compared to ACEi or ARB monotherapy. The first-in-class ARNI represented by a combination of sacubitril and valsartan demonstrated superior efficacy compared to ACEi or an ARB monotherapy in patients with heart failure, as evidenced in the PARADIGM-HF and PARAGON-HF trials. A comprehensive analysis of these studies revealed that sacubitril/valsartan reduced the risk of serious adverse renal outcomes and decline in eGFR, compared to valsartan or enalapril, irrespective of baseline renal function [23].

But renal advantages of ARNI over monotherapy with renin-angiotensin system (RAS) blockers in patients with heart failure remain a subject of debate. Three observational studies and a small-scale randomized controlled trial (RCT) have produced conflicting results. A *post hoc* analysis of the PARADIGM-HF trial revealed a 21% lesser annual decline in GFR in the sacubitril/valsartan arm compared to the ACEi monotherapy arm, despite a greater increase in albuminuria by 25% in a subset of the study with known albuminuria [24]. A recent retrospective study involving patients with advanced CKD (eGFR<30 ml/min) reported no additional benefit of ARNI over ACEi monotherapy in reducing renal outcomes [25]. In PARAGON-HF trial, ARNI demonstrated a noteworthy 50% reduction in the risk of renal outcomes compared to ARB monotherapy [23]. However, a small RCT involving patients with eGFR 20–60 ml/min/1.73 m^2 did not reveal benefits of ARNI in patients with eGFR <30 ml/min/1.73 m^2 both in the presence and absence of heart failure (HF). Intriguingly, ARNI treatment in patients with end-stage kidney disease (ESKD) showed improvement in echocardiographic (echo) parameters after 1 year of treatment [26]. Moreover, there is a lack of studies evaluating the efficacy of ARNI over ACEi or ARB monotherapy in patients with CKD in the absence of HF. Given this information, it seems reasonable to consider ARNIs over ACEi or ARB monotherapy primarily for reducing cardiovascular events in patients with HF and with cautious use in patients with HF and comorbid CKD. This therapeutic approach should be avoided in individuals at risk of hyperkalemia, particularly in patients with eGFR <30 ml/min/1.73 m^2 and a systolic blood pressure < 110 mmHg. Anticipating a decline in eGFR within 1 month after initiating therapy is prudent, blood pressure should be closely monitored to rule out hypotension, and if necessary, downtitration of other antihypertensive drugs might be required. Currently, there is no indication for utilizing this drug in patients with CKD without HF solely for the purpose of preventing CKD progression [27].

5. Selective mineralocorticoid receptor antagonist

Patients with type 2 diabetic chronic kidney disease are commonly managed with renin-angiotensin-aldosterone system inhibitors (RAASi), SGLT2i, and hypoglycemic agents. Despite the use of ACEi/ARB, these patients often face adverse cardiorenal outcomes. Steroidal mineralocorticoid receptor antagonists (MRAs), such as spironolactone and eplerenone, can be considered in combination with RAASi and SGLT2i, although there are associated risks of side effects, such as acute kidney injury and hyperkalemia, particularly when used concomitantly with ACEi/ARB. A newer nonsteroidal and selective MRA, finerenone, has been introduced, offering a better tolerability compared to traditional MRAs due to intraclass pharmacological differences. Finerenone demonstrates higher potency for anti-inflammatory and antifibrotic effects compared to other MRAs. The FIGARO-DKD trial involved individuals with type 2 diabetes mellitus (type 2 DM) with eGFR 25–90 ml/min/1.73 m^2 and ACR 30–300 mg/g, or with eGFR above 60 ml/min/1.73 m^2 and ACR 300–5000 mg/g. Finerenone exhibited an 18% improvement in the composite cardiovascular outcome. The Finerenone in Reducing Kidney Failure and Disease Progression in Diabetic Kidney Disease (FIDELIO-DKD) trial assessed the efficacy of finerenone in patients with type 2 DM with urinary ACR between 30 and 300 mg/g and eGFR 25–60 ml/min/1.73 m^2, or ACR between 300 and 5000 mg/g and eGFR over 25 ml/min/1.73 m^2. Finerenone reduced the progression of CKD by 18% and the composite cardiovascular outcome by 13%. In a pooled analysis of both trials, finerenone demonstrated a 14–23% reduction in cardiorenal outcomes in patients with type 2 diabetic CKD at risk of incident heart failure [28].

Subgroup analyses indicate that the beneficial effects of finerenone might be more pronounced in patients with baseline CV disease. It should be noted that the eligibility for those studies was based on the tolerability of maximal doses of ACEi/ARB and the serum potassium below 4.8 mmol/l. Following randomization, 18% developed hyperkalemia, 5% experienced AKI and there was an additional drop in mean systolic blood pressure by 3 mmHg accompanied by an acute decline in eGFR at the initiation of finerenone, which subsequently stabilized during follow-up. It is intriguing that in the FIDELIO-DKD trial, 4% of the participants were already on treatment with SGLT2i; however, it remains unclear whether patients already on SGLT2i could benefit from the addition of finerenone. This question is being investigated in the ongoing CONFIDENCE (Combination effect of finerenone and empagliflozin in participants with chronic kidney disease and type 2 diabetes using a UACR endpoint) study that aims to evaluate how effective and safe is this combination [29].

As MRAs are RAAS blockers, the combined use (dual RAAS blockade) raises concerns about potential higher incidence of renal dysfunction, up to dialysis dependence, identified two decades ago. Consequently, the use of finerenone in addition to ACEi/ARB for patients with type 2 diabetes mellitus (DM) and CKD, with an eGFR 25–60 ml/min/1.73 m^2 and microalbuminuria or eGFR 25–75 ml/min/1.73 m^2 and macroalbuminuria, may be justifiable in the absence of hyperkalemia on the previous maximal ACEi/ARB dose. Initiating this treatment requires thorough monitoring for AKI, hypotension, and hyperkalemia, with an expected acute drop in eGFR during the first month of therapy. The potential use of this combination in patients with nephrotic range proteinuria (ACR >5000 mg/g) remains unconfirmed.

It is imperative for nephrologists to adopt a more precise approach, seeking better information solutions that consider inflammatory signals, platelet activation, baseline patient characteristics, metabolic abnormalities, and other advanced CKD disorders. Previous large CV outcome trials recruited participants enriched for CV diseases where CKD was either underrepresented, or excluding those with eGFR <30 ml/min/1.73 m^2.

6. Sodium-glucose transporter 2 inhibitors

The EMPA-KIDNEY study [30] (Empagliflozin in Patients with Chronic Kidney Disease) distinguished itself from comparable previous investigations by having a lower proportion of patients with diabetes mellitus (46%) than without diabetes. Furthermore, the study included a higher representation of individuals with low kidney function and low levels of albuminuria (**Figure 1**).

The study showed that allocation to empagliflozin resulted in a modest initial 2-month dip in kidney function of 2 ml/min/1.73 m^2 (or 6%), followed by a subsequent halving of the decrease rate in chronic phase of study. This overall outcome underscored a notable 29% reduction in the categorical composite outcome (ESKD, a 40% reduction of eGFR to below 10 ml/min/1.73 m^2, or death from kidney failure). Consistent with other trials of SGLT2 inhibitors, the favorable effects of empagliflozin

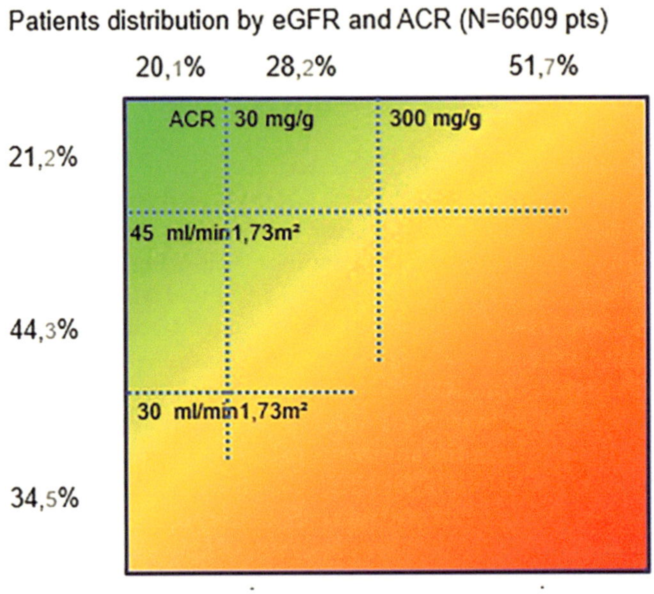

Figure 1.
Patients distribution by kidney function and albuminuria in EMPA-KIDNEY study. Dotted line represent borders of 30 and 300 mg/g in albumin to creatinine ratio in albuminuria distribution, and borders 30 and 45 ml/min/1.73 m² - in eGFR distribution.

on CKD progression exhibited variations based on diabetes status, eGFR, most significantly, albuminuria. The relative effect might be more pronounced in certain populations. The great variety of patients included in the large EMPA-KIDNEY trial facilitated a thorough evaluation of these differences, especially since EMPA-KIDNEY included participants with an eGFR <25 ml/min/1.73 m^2 and with ACR <200 mg/g who were excluded from other trials.

The acute dip in eGFR in EMPA-KIDNEY averaged <3 ml/min/1.73 m^2 or < 10% of baseline eGFR and was more prominent in patients with diabetes, reflecting the higher prevalence and degree of hyperfiltration in DM. The associated rapid reduction in albuminuria supports this hypothesis with the decrease in intraglomerular pressure presumed mechanism of the SGLT2i beneficial effects on kidney function [31]. The secondary analysis of EMPA-KIDNEY suggests that the albuminuria reduction is possibly the most crucial predictor of the benefits, explaining a substantial portion of the effect on significant outcomes [32].

The chronic slope of eGFR is more informative for longer time periods. Although the magnitude of the acute dip correlates with the relative reduction in the chronic slope, measuring the total slope over 2–3 years reduces variation between subgroups. For the objective of delaying kidney failure, it is necessary to consider longer treatment durations. There was no strong evidence that the beneficial effect was significantly modified by the presence or absence of diabetes. Contrary to the KDIGO CKD guidelines (2024) that only suggest (but not definitely recommend) using SGLT2i in patients without diabetes and moderate albuminuria (ACR <200 mg/g), secondary analysis of EMPA-KIDNEY suggests that such patients are likely to gain substantial benefit in terms of preservation of kidney function, in addition to the cardiovascular benefits and reductions in risk of acute kidney injury with longer treatment.

7. Prevention of episodes of acute renal injury

If the effectiveness of pharmacological interventions within the framework of a nephroprotective strategy has not been confirmed for all stages of CKD, the effectiveness of preventing episodes of AKI is beyond doubt under any circumstances. AKI episodes are closely linked with substantial mortality and comorbidity, elevating the risk of compromised renal function. The AKI process, being interconnected, acts as a pathway and catalyst for subsequent AKI episodes and, potentially, the onset of CKD, irrespective of whether renal function is restored following AKI episodes [33]. Biomarkers of AKI play a pivotal role in successfully predicting its development and guiding the selection of interventions for prevention.

8. Nosotropic treatment within the framework of nephroprotection

The etiologies of CKD exert diverse impacts on the progression of kidney disease. Strategies for etiotropic treatment of CKD remain inadequately defined.

Glomerulopathy is a heterogeneous group of diseases and is the cause of a significant number of CKD variants. Despite efforts to find new diagnostic tools, such as "liquid biopsy," for specific markers, kidney biopsy is still the gold standard for diagnosis. Proteinuria exceeding 1 g/day is a risk factor for a rapid decrease in GFR. Certain genetic factors, such as the apolipoprotein L1 (APOL1) genotype in focal segmental glomerulosclerosis or Fabry disease, contribute to accelerated GFR loss. In 2021, KDIGO issued extensive clinical guidelines on glomerular diseases.

Diabetes mellitus is the most widespread etiology of CKD, globally encompassing CKD5. Diabetic nephropathy manifests more often not only in patients with inadequate glycemic control, but it also develops in 30–40% of patients with intensive glycemic control, highlighting the complex and multifactorial pathogenesis of the disease [34]. Alongside optimal glycemic control, SGLT2i and RAAS blockade are central elements in the treatment of diabetic nephropathy. Pentoxifylline and statins exhibit an antiproteinuric effect and decelerate the progression of CKD in patients already receiving RAAS blockers [35].

Chronic kidney disease associated with hypertension ranks among the most prevalent causes of diminished kidney function. While the question of the target blood pressure values and the justified intensity of therapy remains open, blood pressure reduction stands as one of the most crucial strategies in managing patients with hypertension and CKD. Pharmacotherapy, in addition to lifestyle changes, remains indispensable in most cases.

Nephrolithiasis significantly increases the risk of developing CKD and manifesting in 2–3% of CKD5 cases. Patients experiencing stone formation have a lower eGFR, since nephrolithiasis shares several common risk factors with CKD, including nephrotoxic analgesic use, reduced water intake, recurrent infections, structural disorders of the urinary tract, and contrast nephropathy. It is noteworthy that both surgery and shockwave lithotripsy cause damage to the renal parenchyma, inflammation, and fibrosis. Different types of stones correlate with different risks of developing CKD, with the highest risk being cystine, urate, and struvite stones [36].

Autosomal dominant polycystic kidney disease (ADPKD) stands out as the predominant genetic cause of advanced CKD. Traditional nephroprotection has a limited effect on the rate of GFR decrease, so transplantation is the best strategy in this case.

Tolvaptan, a vasopressin-2 receptor (V2R) antagonist, demonstrates efficacy in randomized controlled trials (RCTs) and real-world settings by reducing kidney volume growth from 11–3% and decreasing the GFR decline from 3.3 to 2.3 ml/min/1.73 m^2/year [37]. Importantly, positive GFR dynamics persist, irrespective of variations in total kidney volume growth rates. The incidence of complications, such as elevated liver enzymes, thirst, and hyperuricemia, remains low (7–8% each).

9. Correction of chronic kidney disease syndromes as part of a nephroprotective strategy

Clinical manifestations of CKD vary depending on the etiology, stage, and comorbidity. The kidneys not only provide solute excretion and water-electrolyte balance, but also support endocrine homeostasis. As CKD progresses, these vital functions diminish, leading to the accumulation of uremic toxins. Managing complications arising from CKD not only alleviates associated symptoms but also holds the potential to decelerate the progression of kidney disease.

The incidence of metabolic acidosis rises proportionally with the decline in GFR, heightening the risks of adverse outcomes, including the CKD progression. The implementation of alkylating therapy, such as sodium bicarbonate preparations or dietary measures, proves effective in retarding CKD development [38]. The multifaceted mechanism behind this process may encompass heightened ammonia production in the remaining nephrons, which can lead to the activation of complement with tubulointerstitial lesions and increased endothelin production. Besides renal implications, metabolic acidosis detrimentally impacts cardiovascular outcomes by intensifying inflammatory reactions, boosting aldosterone secretion, and enhancing endothelin synthesis, thereby disrupting contractile ability. Furthermore, metabolic acidosis is linked to impaired bone mineralization, insulin resistance, and overall elevation in all-cause mortality [35].

The exploration of erythropoiesis-stimulating drugs to correct anemia and potentially confer nephroprotection has been ongoing for years. The theoretical nephroprotective effect of these drugs could stem from mitigating renal hypoxia or activating pleiotropic mechanisms. Studies have identified erythropoietin receptors in the mesangium, proximal tubules, and cells of medullary collecting tubules. However, attempts to fully correct anemia did not lead to any benefit and may have caused harm [39]. A decade after the Trial to Reduce Cardiovascular Events with Aranesp Therapy (TREAT) and Correction of Hemoglobin in Outcomes and Renal Insufficiency (CHOIR) studies, efforts were again made to impede the CKD progression with low doses of long-acting erythropoietin drugs in patients without anemia or diabetes mellitus with the previous high target hemoglobin levels of 110–130 g/l, but these efforts were unsuccessful [40, 41]. Nevertheless, there is consensus on the efficacy of correcting anemia from low levels to the target range defined by current clinical recommendations [35]. Phase III registration studies have not confirmed the theoretical possibility of slowing the progression of CKD with the use of hypoxia-induced factor stabilizers. The optimal timing for the use of these drugs during CKD progression may be a crucial factor in achieving the desired effect [42].

The association of hyperuricemia with higher rates of CKD progression has been consistently confirmed over an extended period. However, the ability of hypouricemic drugs to impede the CKD progression by reducing the uric acid levels is less unequivocal. A systematic analysis of randomized controlled trials in 2022 [43] concluded that topiroxostat significantly improved eGFR and reduced ACR. While febuxostat did not exhibit an overall positive effect, it significantly improved renal function (eGFR) in a subgroup of patients with CKD and hyperuricemia. Conversely, allopurinol and pegloticase did not demonstrate a positive effect. Dietary efforts to limit uric acid intake appear reasonable in any case.

10. Evaluation of CKD progression by surrogate criteria

The predictive utility of the GFR reduction curve slope in anticipating robust clinical outcomes was scrutinized in a comprehensive meta-analysis encompassing 47 RCTs with 11 distinct interventions [44]. The meta-regression analysis revealed that each 0.75 ml/min/1.73 m^2/increase in treatment effect on the overall GFR slope was associated with an average risk reduction of 27% (95% CI 20–34%) in hard clinical outcomes. Across the 47 studies involving 60,000 patients, the average eGFR stood at 62 ± 26 ml/min/1.73 m^2 with a median albuminuria of 60 mg/g. The combined average total slope for all studies over 3 years was −3.49 (95% CI–4.04 ÷ −2.93) ml/min/1.73 m^2/year in the control group and − 2.94 (95% CI–3.45 ÷ −2.43) ml/min/1.73 m^2/year in the treatment group. In another meta-analysis [45] involving 41 RCTs with nearly 30,000 participants, the cumulative clinical endpoint was reached by 13% of patients over a median duration of 3.4 years.

In meta-regression analysis, a notable 30% reduction in the geometric mean value of albuminuria resulting from treatment, when compared with the control group, demonstrated an associated average decrease of 27% in the risk of reaching hard clinical endpoints. This correlation exhibited further enhancement when the analysis was confined to patients with baseline albuminuria exceeding 30 mg/g. Consequently, alterations in albuminuria can serve as a meaningful surrogate endpoint for gauging the progression of CKD, especially in patients with high baseline albuminuria. Another meta-analysis, involving 28 cohorts comprising 700,000 participants in observational studies, underscored the significance of a 30% reduction in albuminuria, linking it to a substantial 22% decrease in the risk of advancing to ESKD (95% CI 34 ÷ 8%) [46].

The existing approach to managing patients with late-stage CKD is deemed suboptimal, lacking the necessary correction for pivotal uremic syndromes and exacerbating the likelihood of subsequent prolonged dialysis treatment. Previous publications by the authors outlined the conventional practice for managing late-stage CKD patients [47, 48]. Comparing its results with the results of the implementation of the intensive follow-up program in a prospective study, we assessed the importance of the program components in the "transition center" model.

11. Single center experience of renoprotection on CKD3B-5 stages

The effectiveness of conventional nephroprotection is reduced in the late stages of CKD; the search for effective algorithms is hampered by accelerating decline in glomerular filtration rate. The absence of universally accepted methods for evaluating the effectiveness of conventional nephroprotection prompted our two-year study, aimed at constructing a predictive model for the glomerular filtration decline rate. This model served as a tool to assess the effectiveness of intensive follow-up strategies.

From the city's comprehensive database (n = 7696), we carefully selected a representative group undergoing regular follow-up (n = 540) to build the model predicting the annual glomerular filtration decline rate. This model is used to evaluate the effectiveness of intensive monitoring in the target group of patients (n = 100) with CKD3B-5 using the difference between predicted and actual glomerular filtration rate decline. A matched subgroup (n = 200) was utilized for a direct comparison of both hard and surrogate outcomes.

Patients in the advanced stages of CKD are at significant risk of early mortality, comorbidities, and declines in physical and mental functions as the disease progresses. These risks compete with the risk of developing the need for renal replacement therapy (RRT). The classical concepts of nephroprotective therapy aimed at improving intrarenal hemodynamics with the exception of hyperfiltration [3] are currently complemented by a set of measures that can slow down the decline in renal function, which simultaneously reduces the risks of the development and manifestations of renal insufficiency syndromes. To assess the effectiveness of these interventions, often administered concurrently, operational tools are needed that do not involve a long waiting for results. This prompts the pertinent question within the nephrology community: "Is it right to wait for dialysis to evaluate nephroprotective therapy?" [49].

The intensive follow-up program, integral to our study, involved a heightened frequency of visits—every 2–3 months for CKD3B, every 2 months for CKD4, and monthly for CKD5, with increased frequency as deemed necessary, including remote consultations. During the visit, clinical and laboratory assessments were carried out with the measurement of eGFR using the Chronic Kidney Disease Epidemiology Collaboration (CKD-EPI) formula, as well as proteinuria assessment. In cases of eGFR uncertainty, GFR was directly measured (average value between renal creatinine/urea clearances). Quarterly assessments included parathyroid hormone, ferritin, magnesium, and urate levels, while vitamin D and lipid spectrum evaluations were conducted semiannually. Echocardiography (echo), ultrasound (US) examination, and densitometry were performed once and, if necessary, repeatedly. The Charlson Comorbidity Index (CCI) assessed comorbidity, and additional interventions, such as bioimpedance, consultations with vascular surgeons and psychologists, and scintigraphy/ultrasound examinations of the parathyroid glands, were conducted based on indications. Joint decision about the time of RRT start and the chosen method was made, with due consideration for the feasibility of living donor transplantation. Vaccinations against hepatitis B and pneumococcus were administered as required. The key interventions are detailed in **Table 1**.

The recruitment process for the treatment group was nonselective, encompassing all consecutively admitted patients for follow-up with CKD3B or higher. The control group, intended for assessing advanced CKD progression under standard care, comprised 540 patients with regular follow-up (at least five visits annually). Among these, 200 patients were meticulously matched with the intensive care group based on gender, age, and primary diagnosis. The initiation of follow-up for each pair of patients in control group was attributed to the eGFR level of the matched patient from the intensive care group. For the majority of patients (72%), individual eGFR reduction trajectories were best described by a polynomial function corresponding to the acceleration of eGFR decline:

$$eGFR = -0.0078 \times x^2 + 0.8377 + 11.98 \quad (1)$$

where x – time till actual or potential RRT need (10 ml/min/1.73 m^2).

Intervention	Details
Implementing lifestyle modifications	Incorporating physical activity, achieving weight normalization, and promoting smoking cessation.
Limiting salt intake	For individual patients, monitoring daily sodium excretion and assessing water volumes through bioimpedance.
Limiting protein intake to 0.6–0.8 g/kg/day	In specific patients, monitoring daily urea excretion, supplemented with ketoanalogues of amino acids, aiming for a protein intake of less than 0.6 g/kg/day.
Limiting potassium intake or addressing potassium deficiency	Monitoring is essential when prescribing or adjusting doses of RAAS blockers, diuretics, and mineralocorticoid receptor antagonists, with particular attention to "life-saving therapy" involving potassium sorbents
Prescription of RAAS blockers when proteinuria exceeds 1 g/day (if not prescribed previously)	Assessment of the Renin-Angiotensin-Aldosterone System (RAAS) effectiveness in reducing proteinuria, monitored alongside creatinine levels and potassium dynamics.
Prescribing or adjusting antihypertensive therapy	Aiming for a target blood pressure below 140/90 mmHg or tailored to individual needs
Adjusting phosphatemia to values below 1.45 mmol/l, achieving calcemia within the target range of 2.15–2.5 mmol/l, and managing hyperparathyroidism within the target range based on CKD stages	Implementing a dietary regimen, reducing excessive inorganic phosphate load, utilizing phosphate binders, and managing secondary hyperparathyroidism through vitamin D and alfacalcidol (paricalcitol).
Correction anemia to achieve a hemoglobin target level of 110–120 g/l	Administering intravenous iron when ferritin levels are below 100 mcg/l and C-reactive protein is less than 5 mg/l, subsequently prescribing erythropoietin
Rectifying acidosis to achieve a standard bicarbonate level of 22 mmol/l or higher	Oral administration of sodium bicarbonate, coupled with dietary measures
Prescribing statins for individuals at high risk of cardiovascular events	In accordance with the KDIGO CKD guidelines
Prescribing SGLT2 inhibitors	Collaborative decision-making involving an endocrinologist
Correcting magnesium deficiency	Exclusion of hypermagnesemia
Feasible correction of the inflammatory state	Incorporating dental consultation

Table 1.
The program of intensive follow-up.

The overall rates of eGFR decline were – 2,76 (–3,26÷ – 2,36) for CKD3B, –4,34 (–5,01÷ – 3,46) for CKD4, and – 6,01 (–7,11÷ – 5,23) ml/min/1.73 m^2/year for CKD5.

To predict the "instantaneous" rate of GFR decrease, the calculation of the first derivatives of each of the nonlinear functions was employed. The obtained forecasts of the rate of decrease were then compared with the actual rates of the GFR decrease of each patient. The standard deviation for the models was 0.467, 0.472, 1.046, and 1.763 ml/min/1.73 m^2/year, respectively, when using polynomial, power, logarithmic, and linear functions. The optimal curve approximating this set is:

$$\Delta(eGFR) = -0.0007\times(eGFR)^2 + 0.0155\times(eGFR) + 0.738 \qquad (2)$$

where $\Delta(eGFR)$ is the month rate of GFR decrease and *eGFR* is the current level of GFR. This equation predicts the rate of eGFR decrease by its actual level for the group of regular care (n = 540). The uncertainty, associated with factors other than the level of renal function, decreases with GFR lowering and for eGFR 20–10 ml/min/1.73 m^2 does not exceed 10%.

According to the model developed (in the standard follow-up group), the predicted rate of GFR decline was calculated for each patient in the intensive follow-up group. The predicted values were then compared with the actual rates of CKD progression. The predicted value was 9.06 ± 0.59 ml/min/1.73 m^2/year, while the actual value was 5.98 ± 1.69 ml/min/1.73 m^2/year. This indicates that in the intensive follow-up group, the real rate of GFR decrease was less than the forecast by 3.09 ± 1.92 ml/min/1.73 m^2/year (i.e., by 34 ± 19%).

In the multiple regression analysis with the dependent variable "annual rate of GFR decrease," the association of CKD progression rate with various factors in the intensive follow-up group (n = 100) was estimated (**Table 2**).

As a result of nephroprotective measures, many parameters have been improved that affect the prognosis of patients' survival, the development of cardiovascular complications, and manifestations of uremic syndrome, as well as the progression of CKD (**Table 3**).

To ascertain the comparative impact of interventions, a multiple regression analysis was conducted, with the dependent variable being "the effect of intensive follow-up on the reduction in the rate of eGFR decrease," that is, the size of reduction in the

Regression parameter	**B**	**SD(B)**	**p**	**95%CI for B**
Constant	−4.026	2.111	0.06	−8.22÷ + 0.168
Systolic blood pressure (per 5 mmHg)	−0.145	0.04	0.0005	−0.045÷ − 0.013
Phosphates (per 0.2 mmol/l)	−0.13	0.04	0.001	−1.052÷ − 0.269
Hemoglobin (per 1 g/dl)	0.14	0.07	0.055	−0.0003÷ + 0.028
Albumin (per 1.5 g/l)	0.146	0.057	0.012	0.034÷0.257
Urates (per 0.1 mmol/l)	−0.137	0.064	0.034	−2.637÷ − 0.103
Deviation of the calcium level (0.1 mmol/l from the target)	−0.150	0.076	0.052	−3.004÷ + 0.012
Proteinuria (per 0.1 g/l)	−0.146	0.067	0.032	−2.783÷ − 0.126
Standard bicarbonate (per 2 mmol/l)	0.153	0.067	0.022	0.011÷0.142
The final GFR (per 1 ml/min/1.73 m^2)	0.132	0.029	>0.0001	0.074÷0.19
Initial GFR (per 2 ml/min/1.73 m^2)	−0.134	0.042	0.002	−0.11÷ − 0.025
Diagnosis (for one category in sequential list*)	−0.247	0.054	>0.0001	−0.353÷ − 0.14

**The diagnoses are arranged in order of increasing average eGFR decline rate.*

Table 2.
Model of multivariate regression analysis with a dependent variable "annual rate of glomerular filtration rate decline" (n = 100).

Parameter	Baseline	During treatment	Difference in paired comparisons, p	
Administration of RAAS blockers* for proteinuria of more than 1 g/day or hypertension, without episodes of hyperkalemia (n = 71)				
Proteinuria, Me (Q1–Q3), g/l	0.61 (0.38–1.12)	0.51 (0.27–0.89)	−18% (−0.11; 0.03÷ − 0.24)	<0.001
Creatinine, M ± SD, mmol/l	0.198 ± 0.033	0.234 ± 0.087	+18% (0.04 ± 0.02)	<0.001
Episodes of K+ > 6 mmol/l, n	0/71	4/71	+6%	0.042
Correction of arterial hypertension (n = 51)*				
Mean systolic blood pressure, M ± SD, mmHg	151 ± 7	140 ± 8	−8 ± 6	<0.001
Proportion of patients with hypertension, n (%)	51/100 (51%)	20/100 (20%)	31 reached normal BP	<0.001
Correction of anemia** (at baseline hemoglobin <100 g/l (n = 21)				
Hemoglobin, M ± SD, g/dl	9.6 ± 0.3	11.1 ± 1.1	+1.4 ± 0.7	<0.001
Ferritin#, Me (Q1–Q3), mcg/l	17 (13–44)	104 (88–243)	89 (74–176)	<0.001
Transferrin saturation, M ± SD	18 ± 4%	22 ± 6%	+3 ± 5%	=0.012
Correction of protein and energy wasting**				
Albumin (at baseline <3.5 g/dl), M ± SD, g/l (n = 32)	3.2 ± 0.2	3.4 ± 0.3	+0.2 ± 0.2	<0.001
Transferrin (at baseline <2 g/l), M ± SD, g/L (n = 36)	1.69 ± 0.29	1.86 ± 0.38	+0.16 ± 0.36	0.012
Lymphocytes (at baseline <2.0 × 109/L), M ± SD, (n = 31)	1.48 ± 0.31	1.88 ± 0.32	+0.39 ± 0.52	<0.001
Correction of mineral and bone disorders				
Phosphates* (at baseline >1.13 mmol/l), M ± SD, n = 77)	1.73 ± 0.42	1.53 ± 0.29	−0.21 ± 0.18	<0.001
Calcium* (at baseline >2.5 mmol/l), M ± SD, (n = 28)	2.66 ± 0.08	2.51 ± 0.10	−0.14 ± 0.11	<0.001
Calcium* (at baseline <2.1 mmol/L), M ± SD, (n = 34)	1.97 ± 0.09	2.12 ± 0.11	+0.16 ± 0.13	<0.001
Parathyroid hormone** (at baseline >70 pg./ml) (n = 56), Me (Q1–Q3), pg./ml	174; 79–380	87; 36–209	−140 (−2... − 278)	<0.001
25(OH)D3***, normal/insufficiency/ deficiency	9%/62%/29%	18%/79%/3%	shift towards normal	<0.001
Counteraction to inflammatory state***				
Exacerbation of chronic inflammatory diseases*	11/100	6/100		0.205
The necessary sanitation of the oral cavity			35/78	
C-reactive protein* (at baseline >5 mg/l) (n = 34), Me (Q1–Q3)	8 (6–14)	6 (4–11)	-2 (−3... + 1)	0.023

Parameter	Baseline	During treatment	Difference in paired comparisons, p	
Correction of acid-base state*				
SB* (at baseline <22 mmol/l), M ± SD, (n = 64)	19 ± 2	23 ± 3	+5 ± 3	<0.001
(proportion of patients achieving the goal)			38/64	

**Assessment every visit.*
***Assessment every 3 months.*
****Assessment every 6 months.*
#Without signs of inflammation.

Table 3.
Immediate results of nephroprotective measures.

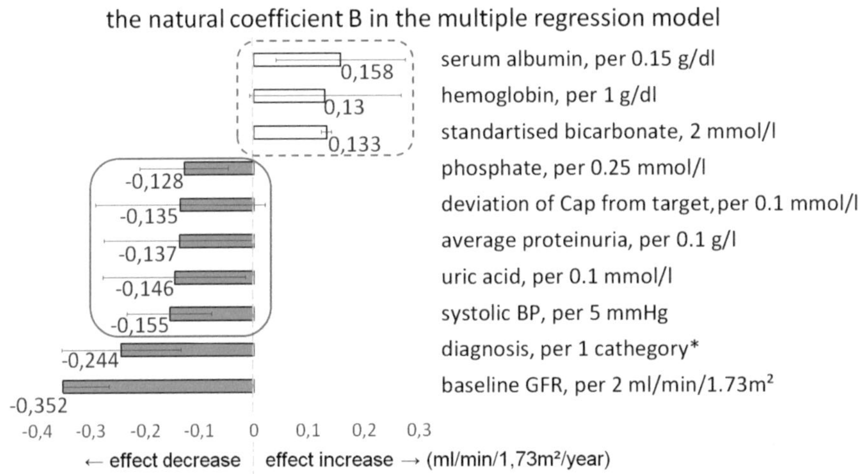

Figure 2.
*A model of multiple regression analysis with a dependent variable "the effect of intensive follow-up on reducing estimated glomerular filtration rate decline"; * - diagnosis ranged in increasing order by average rate of GFR decline.*

actual rate of GFR decline in contrast to the predicted rate. The statistical significance of the model is F = 28.610, p < 0.001 (**Figure 2**).

Each improvement in modifiable positive parameters resulting from interventions (serum albumin by 0.15 g/dl, hemoglobin by 1 g/l, and standard bicarbonate (SB) by 2 mmol/l) or reduction in negative parameters (serum phosphate by 0.25 mmol/l, plasma calcium deviation from target range by 0.1 mmol/l, uric acid by 0.1 mmol/l, systolic blood pressure by 5 mmHg) was independently associated with approximately similar (2.5%) reduction of the rate of GFR decline.

The predicted time to reach the threshold for RRT starting from a conditional point of 20 ml/min/1.73 m^2 for the treatment group was 5.2 ± 1.9 months longer than in the regular follow-up group. Although the average GFR values at the initiation of dialysis were comparable in the treatment group (6.6 ± 1.1 ml/min/1.73 m^2) and the matched group (6.0 ± 1.7 ml/min/1.73 m^2; p = 0.35), its distribution suggested the presence of a delayed and possibly premature start. In the treatment group, the initiation was consistently planned, whereas in the control group, only

58.5% (31/53) of patients commenced dialysis under planned circumstances (χ^2-test; $p < 0.0001$). Notably, in the matched control group, 18.8% (9/53) of patients initiated hemodialysis urgently with a central venous catheter, and in 20.5% (8/39) of cases, initiation with an arteriovenous fistula was necessitated before the lapse of 2 weeks.

12. Discussion

Retrospective studies often concentrate on patients reaching the need for dialysis, with higher progression rates as "progressors" are more likely to necessitate dialysis. In a meta-analysis [50] involving 43 CKD3–4 cohorts and 17 retrospective studies with patients initiating dialysis, annual eGFR decreases were reported as 2.4 (95% CI 2.2–2.6) and 8.5 (95% CI 6.8–10.1) ml/min/1.73 m^2, respectively. Notably, only 4 out of 60 studies, including our present study, explored the nonlinearity of CKD progression. The predominant assumption of linearity in GFR reduction rates in many studies masks potential nonlinearity. Standard care in advanced CKD does not effectively impede CKD progression, surpassing the rates observed in some studies [50], with considerable variations across populations. Urgent dialysis initiation is prevalent in large registers, a situation deemed unsatisfactory [51].

The proposed model of CKD progression makes it possible to predict the rate of eGFR reduction in the conditions of standard nephrology care for CKD3–5. The currently recommended by the European Renal Best Practice (ERBP) and International Society of Nephrology (ISN) the Kidney Failure Risk Equation [52] model for four or eight variables suggests the risk calculation of developing a need for RRT after 2 or 5 years (as a percentage). The model favorably differs from the presented one by including several additional parameters, but proceeds from a linear rate of progression. Predicting only the risk of RRT needs development over a certain period of time, the model of N. Tangri et al. cannot evaluate the results of nephroprotective interventions.

In a brief review, we presented the current landscape of nephroprotective interventions in advanced CKD. While individual components show varying degrees of confirmation, their combined effects and real-world application conditions are not considered in detail, and currently there is no generally accepted approach. The Remission Clinic concept (combined almost two decades ago), incorporating classical nephroprotective approaches, demonstrates effectiveness and continues to expand [53]. Few pragmatic studies have been published covering a significant number of interventions [54], although in recent years several groups of drugs have been increasingly evaluated and compared (sometimes in *post hoc* analysis), even in moderate to severe chronic kidney disease [55]. At the same time, the relative contribution of individual components and their real-world impacts require further analysis, considering potential population variations. Our implemented follow-up program achieves significant improvements in clinically relevant surrogate and hard outcomes for advanced CKD patients, as assessed through multiple regression analysis (**Figure 2**).

In the treatment group, the need for RRT has been postponed, and conditions for a "healthy" dialysis start have been provided: only with permanent dialysis access, most of the patients chose peritoneal dialysis, all patients started with targeted eGFR showcasing better correction of anemia, phosphatemia, and calcemia, as well as arterial hypertension. The predicted time to achieve the need for RRT from 20 ml/min/1.73 m^2 in the treatment group was 5 months longer. Thus, in real practice, the accuracy of previous simulation modeling has been confirmed: the predicted lengthening of the predialysis stage of treatment was 1.6 ± 1.7 years (p = 0.002) from the baseline GFR level of 20–40 ml/min/1.73 m^2 [56].

The search for new drugs and methods to slow down the progression of CKD continues intensively.

Interventions aimed at enhancing the elimination of uremic toxins, fluids, and electrolytes from the intestine, as well as the modulation of the intestinal microbiota, may represent new therapeutic strategies for the treatment of uremia in patients with CKD [57].

Although fibrosis can play a protective role, under certain circumstances, it can gradually turn into an uncontrolled irreversible and self-sustaining process. Several systems, molecules, and reactions are involved in the pathogenesis of pathological fibrosis in chronic kidney disease (CKD) such as: inflammation, renin-angiotensin system, parathyroid hormone, fibroblast growth factor 23 (FGF23), Klotho, microRNA (miRNA), and the vitamin D system. These key factors can control/exacerbate fibrosis, having a great effect on the kidneys and heart in CKD [58]. A number of clinical and preclinical studies on the prevention of renal fibrosis are ongoing now [59]. Doubtless, new opportunities will become available in the near future, in particular in relation to patients with advanced CKD stages.

The limitation of this study is the small number (n = 100) of patients in the treatment group, but the developed algorithm continues to be used in real-world practice, and ongoing recruitment of patients with an extended period of active follow-up will reduce the effect of this restriction. Validation of eGFR decrease in rate prediction internally and externally is planned as part of ongoing work in similar programs across different centers.

13. Conclusion

Assessing the rate of GFR decline serves as a valuable method not only for gauging the progression of CKD and predicting the timing of RRT, but also for promptly characterizing intervention outcomes. It is essential to consider the variability and nonlinear nature of the GFR reduction. To reliably evaluate this rate in each patient, utilizing five or more time-spaced eGFR values is recommended. The proposed algorithm of intensive follow-up in the advanced CKD demonstrates the capability to reduce the rate of eGFR decline by a third compared to standard care results. This reduction contributes to mitigating the risks of mortality, delaying the requirement for RRT, and enhancing the correction of uremic syndrome—significant factors in CKD progression.

Acknowledgements

I thank my mother Helena for her support and love, invaluable in my life.

Conflict of interest

The author declares no conflict of interest.

Author details

Daria Sergeevna Sadovskaya
North-Western State Medical University named after I.I. Mechnikov, Russia

*Address all correspondence to: sadovskaya.nephrologist@gmail.com

References

[1] GBD Chronic Kidney Disease Collaboration. Global, regional, and national burden of chronic kidney disease, 1990-2017: A systematic analysis for the global burden of disease study 2017. Lancet. 2020;**395**(10225):709-733. DOI: 10.1016/S0140-6736(20)30045-3

[2] Ramspek CL, Boekee R, Evans M, et al. EQUAL study investigators. Predicting kidney failure, cardiovascular disease and death in advanced CKD patients. Kidney International Reports. 2022;**7**(10):2230-2241. DOI: 10.1016/j.ekir.2022.07.165

[3] Kidney Disease: Improving Global Outcomes (KDIGO) CKD Work Group. KDIGO 2024 Clinical Practice Guideline for the Evaluation and Management of Chronic Kidney Disease. Kidney International. 2024;**105**(4S):S117-S314

[4] Dasgupta I, Zoccali C. Is the KDIGO systolic blood pressure target <120 mm Hg for chronic kidney disease appropriate in routine clinical practice? Hypertension. 2022;**79**(1):4-11. DOI: 10.1161/HYPERTENSIONAHA.121.18434

[5] Kurasawa S, Yasuda Y, Kato S, REACH-J CKD collaborators. Relationship between the lower limit of systolic blood pressure target and kidney function decline in advanced chronic kidney disease: An instrumental variable analysis from the REACH-J CKD cohort study. Hypertension Research. 2023;**46**(11):2478-2487. DOI: 10.1038/s41440-023-01358-z

[6] Zhang F, Bai Y, Zhao X, et al. Therapeutic effects of exercise interventions for patients with chronic kidney disease: An umbrella review of systematic reviews and meta-analyses. BMJ Open. 2022;**12**(9):e054887. DOI: 10.1136/bmjopen-2021-054887

[7] Moriconi D, Antonioli L, Masi S, et al. Glomerular hyperfiltration in morbid obesity: Role of the inflammasome signalling. Nephrology (Carlton, Vic.). 2022;**27**(8):673-680. DOI: 10.1111/nep.14077

[8] Abdul Wahab R, Cohen RV, le Roux CW. Recent advances in the treatment of patients with obesity and chronic kidney disease. Annals of Medicine. 2023;**55**(1):2203517. DOI: 10.1080/07853890.2023.2203517

[9] McMahon EJ, Campbell KL, Bauer JD, et al. Altered dietary salt intake for people with chronic kidney disease. Cochrane Database of Systematic Reviews. 2021;**6**(6):CD010070. DOI: 10.1002/14651858.CD010070.pub3

[10] Naber T, Purohit S. Chronic kidney disease: Role of diet for a reduction in the severity of the disease. Nutrients. 2021;**13**(9):3277. DOI: 10.3390/nu13093277

[11] Komaba H et al. Parathyroidectomy vs cinacalcet among patients undergoing hemodialysis. The Journal of Clinical Endocrinology and Metabolism. 2022;**107**(7):2016-2025. DOI: 10.1210/clinem/dgac142

[12] Tan J, Zhou H, Deng J, at al. Effectiveness of microecological preparations for improving renal function and metabolic profiles in patients with chronic kidney disease. Frontiers in Nutrition. 2022;**9**:850014. DOI: 10.3389/fnut.2022.850014

[13] Fazelian S, Moradi F, Agah S, et al. Effect of omega-3 fatty acids

supplementation on cardio-metabolic and oxidative stress parameters in patients with chronic kidney disease: A systematic review and meta-analysis. BMC Nephrology. 2021;**22**(1):160. DOI: 10.1186/s12882-021-02351-9

[14] Fotheringham AK, Gallo LA, Borg DJ, Forbes JM. Advanced glycation end products (AGEs) and chronic kidney disease: Does the modern diet age the kidney? Nutrients. 2022;**14**(13):2675. DOI: 10.3390/nu14132675

[15] Jiang Z, Wang Y, Zhao X, et al. Obesity and chronic kidney disease. American Journal of Physiology. Endocrinology and Metabolism. 2023;**324**(1):E24-E41. DOI: 10.1152/ajpendo.00179.2022

[16] Xie X, Liu Y, Perkovic V, et al. Renin-angiotensin system inhibitors and kidney and cardiovascular outcomes in patients with CKD: A Bayesian network meta-analysis of randomized clinical trials. American Journal of Kidney Diseases. 2016;**67**(5):728-741. DOI: 10.1053/j.ajkd.2015.10.011

[17] Boggia J, Silvariño R, Ferreiro Fuentes A. Tobacco use and the kidney: A review of public policies and studies on kidney disease progression. Contributions to Nephrology. 2021;**199**:188-200. DOI: 10.1159/000517726

[18] Fu EL, Clase CM, Evans M, et al. Comparative effectiveness of renin-angiotensin system inhibitors and calcium channel blockers in individuals with advanced CKD: A nationwide observational cohort study. American Journal of Kidney Diseases. 2021;**77**(5):719-729.e1. DOI: 10.1053/j.ajkd.2020.10.006

[19] Fu EL, Evans M, Clase CM, et al. Stopping renin-angiotensin system inhibitors in patients with advanced CKD and risk of adverse outcomes: A nationwide study. Journal of the American Society of Nephrology. 2021;**32**(2):424-435. DOI: 10.1681/ASN.2020050682

[20] Kidney Disease: Improving Global Outcomes (KDIGO) Blood Pressure Work Group. KDIGO 2021 clinical practice guideline for the management of blood pressure in chronic kidney disease. Kidney International. 2021;**99**(3S):S1-S87. DOI: 10.1016/j.kint.2020.11.003

[21] Taylor KS, Mclellan J, Verbakel JY, et al. Effects of antihypertensives, lipid-modifying drugs, glycaemic control drugs and sodium bicarbonate on the progression of stages 3 and 4 chronic kidney disease in adults: A systematic review and meta-analysis. BMJ Open. 2019;**9**(9):e030596. DOI: 10.1136/bmjopen-2019-030596

[22] Zhang Y, He D, Zhang W, et al. ACE inhibitor benefit to kidney and cardiovascular outcomes for patients with non-dialysis chronic kidney disease stages 3-5: A network meta-analysis of randomised clinical trials. Drugs. 2020;**80**(8):797-811. DOI: 10.1007/s40265-020-01290-3

[23] Mc, Causland FR, Lefkowitz MP, Claggett B, et al. Angiotensin-neprilysin inhibition and renal outcomes in heart failure with preserved ejection fraction. Circulation. 2020;**142**(13):1236-1245. DOI: 10.1161/CIRCULATIONAHA.120.047643

[24] Damman K, Gori M, Claggett B, et al. Renal effects and associated outcomes during angiotensin-neprilysin inhibition in heart failure. JACC Heart Failure. 2018;**6**(6):489-498. DOI: 10.1016/j.jchf.2018.02.004

[25] Hsiao FC, Lin CP, Yu CC, et al. Angiotensin receptor-neprilysin inhibitors

in patients with heart failure with reduced ejection fraction and advanced chronic kidney disease: A retrospective multi-institutional study. Frontiers in Cardiovascular Medicine. 2022;**9**:794707. DOI: 10.3389/fcvm.2022.794707

[26] Niu CY, Yang SF, Ou SM, et al. Sacubitril/valsartan in patients with heart failure and concomitant end-stage kidney disease. Journal of the American Heart Association. 2022;**11**(18):e026407. DOI: 10.1161/JAHA.122.026407

[27] Tushar Tarun T, Ghanta SN, Vincz Ong V, et al. Updates on new therapies for patients with CKD. Kidney International Reports. 2023;**9**:16-28. DOI: 10.1016/j.ekir.2023.10.006

[28] Agarwal R, Filippatos G, Pitt B, et al. FIDELIO-DKD and FIGARO-DKD investigators. Cardiovascular and kidney outcomes with finerenone in patients with type 2 diabetes and chronic kidney disease: The FIDELITY pooled analysis. European Heart Journal. 2022;**43**(6):474-484. DOI: 10.1093/eurheartj/ehab777

[29] Green JB, Mottl AK, Bakris G, et al. Design of the COmbinatioN effect of FInerenone anD EmpagliflooziN in participants with chronic kidney disease and type 2 diabetes using a UACR endpoint study (CONFIDENCE). Nephrology, Dialysis, Transplantation. 2023;**38**(4):894-903. DOI: 10.1093/ndt/gfac198

[30] EMPA-KIDNEY Collaborative Group; Herrington WG, Staplin N, Wanner C, Green JB, Hauske SJ, Emberson JR, et al. Empagliflozin in Patients with Chronic Kidney Disease. The New England Journal of Medicine. 12 Jan 2023;**388**(2):117-127. DOI: 10.1056/NEJMoa2204233

[31] Jongs N, Greene T, Chertow GM, et al. DAPA-CKD trial committees and investigators. Effect of dapagliflozin on urinary albumin excretion in patients with chronic kidney disease with and without type 2 diabetes: A prespecified analysis from the DAPA-CKD trial. The Lancet Diabetes and Endocrinology. 2021;**9**(11):755-766. DOI: 10.1016/S2213-8587(21)00243-6

[32] EMPA-KIDNEY Collaborative Group. Effects of empagliflozin on progression of chronic kidney disease: A prespecified secondary analysis from the EMPA-KIDNEY trial. The Lancet Diabetes and Endocrinology. 2024;**12**(1):39-50. DOI: 10.1016/S2213-8587(23)00321-2

[33] Lameire NH, Levin A, Kellum JA, et al. Harmonizing acute and chronic kidney disease definition and classification: Report of a kidney disease: Improving global outcomes (KDIGO) consensus conference. Kidney International. 2021;**100**(3):516-526. DOI: 10.1016/j.kint.2021.06.028

[34] Heyman SN, Raz I, Dwyer JP, et al. Diabetic proteinuria revisited: Updated physiologic perspectives. Cell. 2022;**11**(18):2917. DOI: 10.3390/cells11182917

[35] Yan MT, Chao CT, Lin SH. Chronic kidney disease: Strategies to retard progression. International Journal of Molecular Sciences. 2021;**22**(18):10084. DOI: 10.3390/ijms221810084

[36] Uribarri J. Chronic kidney disease and kidney stones. Current Opinion in Nephrology and Hypertension. 2020;**29**(2):237-242. DOI: 10.1097/MNH.0000000000000582

[37] Horie S, Muto S, Kawano H, et al. Preservation of kidney function irrelevant of total kidney volume growth rate with tolvaptan treatment in patients with autosomal dominant

polycystic kidney disease. Clinical and Experimental Nephrology. 2021;**25**(5):467-478. DOI: 10.1007/s10157-020-02009-0

[38] Navaneethan SD, Shao J, Buysse J, Bushinsky DA. Effects of treatment of metabolic acidosis in CKD: A systematic review and meta-analysis. Clinical Journal of the American Society of Nephrology. 2019;**14**(7):1011-1020. DOI: 10.2215/CJN.13091118

[39] Pfeffer MA, Burdmann EA, Chen CY, et al. A trial of darbepoetin alfa in type 2 diabetes and chronic kidney disease. The New England Journal of Medicine. 2009;**361**(21):2019-2032. DOI: 10.1056/NEJMoa0907845

[40] Hayashi T, Maruyama S, Nangaku M, et al. PREDICT investigators. Darbepoetin Alfa in patients with advanced CKD without diabetes: Randomized, controlled trial. Clinical Journal of the American Society of Nephrology. 2020;**15**(5):608-615. DOI: 10.2215/CJN.08900719

[41] Tsuruya K, Hayashi T, Yamamoto H, et al. RADIANCE-CKD study investigators. Renal prognoses by different target hemoglobin levels achieved by epoetin beta pegol dosing to chronic kidney disease patients with hyporesponsive anemia to erythropoiesis-stimulating agent: A multicenter open-label randomized controlled study. Clinical and Experimental Nephrology. 2021;**25**(5):456-466. DOI: 10.1007/s10157-020-02005-4

[42] Miao M, Wu M, Li Y, Zhang L, et al. Clinical potential of hypoxia inducible factors prolyl hydroxylase inhibitors in treating nonanemic diseases. Frontiers in Pharmacology. 2022;**13**:837249. DOI: 10.3389/fphar.2022.837249

[43] Tsukamoto S, Okami N, Yamada T, et al. Prevention of kidney function decline using uric acid-lowering therapy in chronic kidney disease patients: A systematic review and network meta-analysis. Clinical Rheumatology. 2022;**41**(3):911-919. DOI: 10.1007/s10067-021-05956-5

[44] Inker LA, Heerspink HJL, Tighiouart H, et al. GFR slope as a surrogate end point for kidney disease progression in clinical trials: A meta-analysis of treatment effects of randomized controlled trials. Journal of the American Society of Nephrology. 2019;**30**(9):1735-1745. DOI: 10.1681/ASN.2019010007

[45] Heerspink HJL, Greene T, Tighiouart H, et al. Chronic kidney disease epidemiology collaboration. Change in albuminuria as a surrogate endpoint for progression of kidney disease: A meta-analysis of treatment effects in randomised clinical trials. The Lancet Diabetes and Endocrinology. 2019;**7**(2):128-139. DOI: 10.1016/S2213-8587(18)30314-0

[46] Coresh J, Heerspink HJL, Sang Y, et al. Chronic kidney disease prognosis consortium and chronic kidney disease epidemiology collaboration. Change in albuminuria and subsequent risk of end-stage kidney disease: An individual participant-level consortium meta-analysis of observational studies. The Lancet Diabetes and Endocrinology. 2019;**7**(2):115-127. DOI: 10.1016/S2213-8587(18)30313-9

[47] Sadovskaya D, Zemchenkov A, Gerasimchuk R, Sabodash A. Chronic kidney disease progression and outcomes among a population with chronic kidney disease stage 3-5. SUN-115. Kidney International Reports. 2020;**5**(3):S248-S249. DOI: 10.1016/j.ekir.2020.02.642

[48] Sadovskaya DS, Vishnevsky KA, Konakova IN, Bakulina NV. The rate of chronic kidney disease progression in advanced stages and the dynamics of the uremic syndrome parameters. Nephrology (Saint-Petersburg). 2022;**26**(4):50-65. DOI: 10.36485/1561-6274-2022-26-4-50-65

[49] Weldegiorgis M, de Zeeuw D, et al. Is chronic dialysis the right hard renal end point to evaluate renoprotective drug effects? Clinical Journal of the American Society of Nephrology. 2017;**12**(10):1595-1600. DOI: 10.2215/CJN.09590916

[50] Hoshino J, Tsunoda R, Nagai K, et al. Comparison of annual eGFR decline among primary kidney diseases in patients with CKD G3b-5: Results from a REACH-J CKD cohort study. Clinical and Experimental Nephrology. 2021;**25**(8):902-910. DOI: 10.1007/s10157-021-02059-y

[51] Tachikart A, Vachey C, Vauchy C, et al. Determinants of urgent start dialysis in a chronic kidney disease cohort followed by nephrologists. BMC Nephrology. 2023;**24**(1):190. DOI: 10.1186/s12882-023-03222-1

[52] Grams ME, Brunskill NJ, Ballew SH, et al. The kidney failure risk equation: Evaluation of novel input variables including eGFR estimated using the CKD-EPI 2021 equation in 59 cohorts. Journal of the American Society of Nephrology. 2023;**34**(3):482-494. DOI: 10.1681/ASN.0000000000000050

[53] Ruggenenti P, Perticucci E, Cravedi P, et al. Role of remission clinics in the longitudinal treatment of CKD. Journal of the American Society of Nephrology. 2008;**19**(6):1213-1224. DOI: 10.1681/ASN.2007090970

[54] Remission Clinic Task Force; Clinical Research Center Aldo e Cele Daccò. The remission clinic approach to halt the progression of kidney disease. Journal of Nephrology. 2011;**24**(3):274-281. DOI: 10.5301/JN.2011.7763

[55] Tsuchida KI, Taneda S, Yokota I, et al. The renoprotective effect of once-weekly GLP-1 receptor agonist dulaglutide on progression of nephropathy in Japanese patients with type 2 diabetes and moderate to severe chronic kidney disease (JDDM67). Journal of Diabetes Investigation. 2022;**13**(11):1834-1841. DOI: 10.1111/jdi.13877

[56] Zemchenkov A, Rumyantsev A, Smirnov AV. The efficacy evaluation of the nephroprotective therapy: Minireview and Saint Petersburg registry data. Nephrology (Saint-Petersburg). 2018;**22**(1):58-68. DOI: 10.24884/1561-6274-2018-22-1-58-68

[57] Sumida K, Lau WL, Kalantar-Zadeh K, Kovesdy CP. Novel intestinal dialysis interventions and microbiome modulation to control uremia. Current Opinion in Nephrology and Hypertension. 2022;**31**(1):82-91. DOI: 10.1097/MNH.0000000000000753

[58] Panizo S, Martínez-Arias L, Alonso-Montes C, et al. Fibrosis in chronic kidney disease: Pathogenesis and consequences. International Journal of Molecular Sciences. 2021;**22**(1):408. DOI: 10.3390/ijms22010408

[59] Huang W, Chen YY, Li ZQ, et al. Recent advances in the emerging therapeutic strategies for diabetic kidney diseases. International Journal of Molecular Sciences. 2022;**23**(18):10882. DOI: 10.3390/ijms231810882

Chapter 9

Novel Potassium Binders for CKD Patients with Hyperkalemia

Randah Dahlan and Ali Alkatheeri

Abstract

Hyperkalemia is defined as a serum or plasma potassium level that is greater than 5.0 or 5.5 mmol/L, and this variation is because the definition of the upper limit of normal level used in research and guidelines is varied. Hyperkalemia is a potentially life-threatening condition that may lead to muscle paralysis, cardiac arrhythmia, and death. It is a common clinical problem seen in patients with chronic kidney disease (CKD), and this is particularly true with the progressive and advanced deterioration of the glomerular filtration rate (GFR). The management of such patients could be a challenge to nephrologists, especially since the therapeutic interventions that are used to slow the progression of CKD may themselves lead to or worsen hyperkalemia. This chapter will discuss the issue of hyperkalemia in CKD patients and will focus on the role of novel potassium binders in the management of such patients.

Keywords: hyperkalemia, potassium binders, potassium, CKD, patiromer, sodium zirconium cyclosilicate

1. Introduction

Potassium is the major intracellular cation, and 98% of the total body potassium is confined to the intracellular space [1]. The ratio between the intracellular and extracellular potassium concentrations is a very important determinant of the cellular membrane potential [2]. Therefore, any disturbance to this ratio may affect the function of the cardiovascular and neuromuscular systems. In general, hyperkalemia develops when there is increased potassium release from cells or reduced urinary potassium excretion. Chronic kidney disease patients are at particular risk of hyperkalemia because of multiple factors [3]. These factors are summarized in **Figure 1**. With the progressive reduction in the GFR, the urinary excretion of potassium is also progressively decreased. Especially when the dietary potassium intake is not restricted. Additionally, patients with CKD tend to have metabolic acidosis, which will lead to a shift of potassium from the intracellular to the extra-cellular space with subsequent hyperkalemia. Renin–angiotensin–aldosterone system inhibitors (RAASi) are commonly used in patients with CKD to slow the progression to end-stage renal disease. However, this comes with the price of increased risk of hyperkalemia, as RAASi therapy will reduce the secretion of aldosterone, thereby impairing the efficiency of urinary potassium excretion. In addition, CKD patients often have comorbidities, such as DM and heart failure, which are frequently associated with

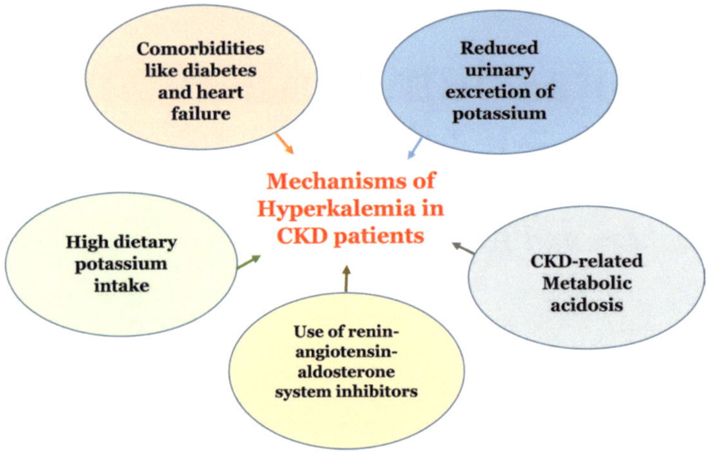

Figure 1.
Mechanisms of hyperkalemia in chronic kidney disease (CKD) patients.

hyperkalemia through different mechanisms [3]. The presence, or even the coexistence, of all aforementioned factors, make hyperkalemia a common encounter for nephrologists when managing CKD patients. This chapter will give a brief overview of the extent of the hyperkalemia problem among CKD patients and its clinical implications but will discuss in detail the role of the novel potassium binders in mitigating the risk of hyperkalemia in patients with CKD.

2. Epidemiology

When looking at the general population, hyperkalemia is most prevalent in patients with CKD [4]. The rate of hyperkalemia among CKD populations is variable depending on multiple factors including the level that was used to define hyperkalemia, the GFR or the stage of CKD, the use of RAASi therapy, and presence of certain comorbidities, such as diabetes and heart failure [5]. Studies focusing on pre-dialysis CKD patients have shown that hyperkalemia is not only common but also recurrent [6–10]. Patients with CKD spend 13–32% of their time in a chronic state of hyperkalemia [9]. In these studies, low GFR seems to be the most important factor associated with hyperkalemia. For example, in a cross-sectional study of pre-dialysis outpatients with an estimated GFR of 14.5 ± 4.8 ml/min/1.73 m^2, the prevalence rate of hyperkalemia, defined as potassium level ≥ 5.0, ≥ 5.5, and ≥ 6.0 mmol/L, was 54.2%, 31.5%, and 8.4%, respectively [7]. In another study of CKD patients with an average GFR of 35.0 ± 17.3 ml/min/1.73 m^2, the prevalence of hyperkalemia was 35.0 ± 17.3% and was dependent on the CKD stage [8]. In the later study, most patients had mild to moderate hyperkalemia (defined as a potassium level of 5.0–5.4 mml/L; and 5.5–5.9 mmol/L, respectively) [8]. Severe hyperkalemia with potassium level ≥ 6.0 mmol/L was rare [8–10].

3. Clinical implications

When encountering patients with hyperkalemia, physicians worry the most about the potential risk of cardiac arrhythmias. However, other consequences of hyperkalemia are also serious [11]. The following summarizes other potential consequences of hyperkalemia observed in patients with CKD:

- *Mortality risk:* Across all CKD stages, hyperkalemia is associated with increased all-cause mortality as well as cardiovascular mortality [12, 13].

- *Hospitalization risk:* The rate of hospitalization related to hyperkalemia is likely the highest in patients with CKD [13]. Some data suggest that hyperkalemia is responsible for more than one-third of total hospitalization in pre-dialysis CKD patients [14]. These hospitalizations could be due to ventricular arrhythmia, cardiac arrest, or other cardiac events [10]

- *A predictor of progression to end-stage renal disease (ESRD):* A multivariable competing-risk analysis of pre-dialysis CKD patients showed that new-onset or persistent hyperkalemia portends per se a 30% higher risk of ESRD, which is independent of the rate of GFR decline [8].

- *Reduction of dose/or cessation of RASSi therapy:* The utilization of RASSi therapy in patients with CKD has been shown to slow the progression of CKD, decrease the risk of cardiovascular events, and decrease the risk of death [15–19]. Additionally, patients with CKD may have co-existing morbidities (like heart diseases), for which RASSi therapy could be beneficial [3]. However, this utilization of RASSi is not always easy or feasible because of the risk of hyperkalemia [3, 20]. Hyperkalemia frequently leads to a reduction of the RASSi dose or even discontinuation in patients with CKD [20–22]. This suboptimal use of RASSI in CKD results in increased rates of death and other major adverse cardiovascular events [20, 22].

- *Other consequences:* neuromuscular abnormalities are seen in patients with CKD, and hyperkalemia could contribute to uremic depolarization and the development of neuropathy [23]. Some data suggest that controlling hyperkalemia may limit the progression of peripheral neuropathy in these patients [24]. Hyperkalemia is also associated with a substantial increase in economic burdens, primarily driven by higher inpatient costs [25].

4. Traditional lines of management

In situations where CKD patients present with a hyperkalemic emergency (e.g., symptomatic hyperkalemia, presence of electrocardiogram (ECG) changes, severe hyperkalemia with a level more than 6.5 mmol/L.... etc.); the usual rapidly acting interventions (i.e., intravenous calcium, salbutamol nebulizer, insulin, and glucose) should be instituted promptly [26]. These interventions are usually followed by therapies that remove potassium from the body, either through the kidneys or through the gastrointestinal tract. However, CKD patients usually have chronic, asymptomatic, mild to moderate hyperkalemia, which may allow for chronic and slowly-acting interventions to be instituted. These traditional interventions are commonly used concomitantly by nephrologists, especially when trying to mitigate the risk of hyperkalemia associated with the use of RASSi therapy. However, all these traditional lines of management have their limitations or possible side effects. For example, CKD patients with hyperkalemia are advised to restrict their dietary potassium intake to 2 to 3 gm per day [26, 27]. However, this approach has many limitations, starting with the fact that CKD patients have many other dietary restrictions which may lead to a high rate of poor compliance [28]. Additionally, strong data to suggest the effectiveness of dietary potassium restriction is lacking [26]. Some data suggest that dietary potassium restriction has the potential to be harmful to overall health and cardiovascular outcomes in such patients [29].

Another example of a common therapeutic intervention for hyperkalemia is the use of sodium polystyrene sulfonate (SPS). SPS is a non-absorbed cation-exchange resin that is sold under the brand names *Kayexalate, SPS, or Kionex* [30]. It was first introduced for the treatment of hyperkalemia in the early 1950s based on 2 small case series and was then approved by the US Food and Drug Administration (FDA) for short-term treatment of hyperkalemia in 1958 [30]. It works by binding to potassium in the colon in exchange for sodium leading to increased fecal excretion of potassium. It is given orally as 15 gm up to 4 times per day or 30–60 gm rectally up to 4 times per day [30, 31]. Although SPS is a famous intervention that has been used for a long time, randomized clinical trials supporting its efficacy for the management of chronic hyperkalemia are limited [30, 32]. There is only one randomized clinical trial with a small sample size of CKD patients which showed that SPS leads to a small reduction in the serum potassium level compared to placebo [30, 32], but the clinical significance of this effect is not clear [30]. Moreover, in 2009, the FDA released a black box warning about the risk of intestinal necrosis (which could be fatal) associated with the use of SPS in combination with sorbitol [30, 32, 33]. However, some data suggests that intestinal necrosis may still occur in patients receiving SPS alone without sorbitol suggesting that this complication is likely related to the SPS itself and independent of sorbitol [30, 34]. Patients with advanced CKD are at particular risk of developing gastrointestinal complications including intestinal ischemia, thrombosis, ulceration, or perforation [35], and the risk of hospitalization because of SPS-related gastrointestinal complications is increased in elderly patients [36]. Looking at all aforementioned concerns about SPS, some have recommended that it should no longer be used [26, 30, 37], or to limit its use to a situation where all the following criteria are met [37]:

- potentially life-threatening hyperkalemia
- Novel potassium binders (i.e., patiromer or sodium zirconium cyclosilicate) are not available,
- dialysis is not readily available, and
- other therapies (like diuretics) have failed or are not possible.

For postoperative patients, patients with intestinal obstruction/ileus, patients with chronic bowel disease, and patients with constipation, hypovolemia, or renal insufficiency, SPS should not be used even in the above-mentioned situation, and such patients can be managed with repeated doses of insulin and glucose until dialysis is feasible [33, 37].

The limitations of traditional lines of management of chronic hyperkalemia before the era of novel potassium binders are summarized in **Table 1**.

Dietary Restriction of Potassium (2 to 3 grams/day)	
Limitations	Patients may already need to follow other dietary restrictions
	Low compliance rate
	Potential Increase in the risk of cardiovascular outcomes and stroke
Loop Diuretics	
Limitations	Its role is mainly in hypervolemic patients
	May cause other electrolyte disturbances and acute kidney injury
	Its efficacy depends on renal function
Sodium Bicarbonate Tablets	
Limitations	Lack of strong evidence to support its role
	Its role is mainly in patients with coexisting metabolic acidosis
	May lead to fluid retention and hypertension
Reduction of Dose /Cessation of Renin– Angiotensin–Aldosterone System Inhibitors	
Limitations	Increase the rate of major adverse cardiovascular events
	Increase the rate of death
	Loss of renoprotective effect of RASSI
Sodium Polystyrene Sulfonate	
Limitations	Rare but serious adverse gastrointestinal side effects
	Limited evidence to support its efficacy, especially as chronic therapy
	May bind other medications reducing their efficacy

Table 1.
Limitations of traditional lines of management of chronic hyperkalemia.

5. Novel potassium binders

The limitations of all the aforementioned interventions in the management of chronic hyperkalemia have identified an unmet need to find a reliable and effective intervention or strategy to address this problem. The introduction of the novel potassium binders has filled a major gap in this regard. In 2015, patiromer was approved by FDA as a novel potassium binder, followed by sodium zirconium cyclosilicate (SZC) which was approved by FDA in 2018. Many trials have demonstrated the efficacy of both drugs in short and long-term management of hyperkalemia [38]. Therefore, many guidelines are now advocating for the use of these novel binders to manage hyperkalemia, especially for those using RASSi therapy [26, 38–40]. **Table 2** compares different potassium binders.

5.1 Patiromer

Patiromer is a cross-linked polymer of 2-fluoroacrylic acid with divinylbenzenes and 1,7-octadiene. It is used in form of its calcium salt and with sorbitol, a combination called patiromer sorbitex calcium.

See **Figure 2**.

Property	Sodium Polystyrene Sulfonate	Patiromer	Sodium Zirconium Cyclosilicate
Brand name	Kayexalate, SPS, or Kionex	Veltassa	Lokelma
Approval year	1958	2015	2018
Mechanism of action	binds potassium in exchange for sodium	binds potassium in exchange for calcium	binds potassium in exchange for sodium and hydrogen
Onset of action	Hours to days	7 hours	1 hour
Site of action	Colon	Distal colon	Entire gastrointestinal tract
Dosing	15–60 g orally (1–4 times daily), or 30–50 g rectally (1–4 times daily)	8.4 g daily, and if needed, may increase the dose after a week to 16.8 g to a maximum of 25.2 g daily	LA: 10 g orally three times daily for 48 hours, then MD: 5 g orally daily. If needed, increase the dose after a week to 10 gm. The maximum dose is 15 g daily
Na content	1500 mg per 15 g	None	400 mg per 5 g
Serious S/E	Colonic necrosis	None	None
Common S/E	• Constipation, diarrhea, nausea, and vomiting • Hypokalemia, hypomagnesemia	• Constipation, diarrhea, nausea, and vomiting • Hypokalemia, hypomagnesemia	• Hypokalemia • Edema
Cost	• 15 g/60 mL (per mL): $1.21	• 8.4 g: $54.77 • 16.8 g: $40.99 • 25.2 g: $40.99	• 5 g: $32.82 • 10 g: $32.82

G: gram, LA: loading dose, MD: maintenance dose, Na: sodium, S/E: side effects.

Table 2.
Comparison of potassium binders.

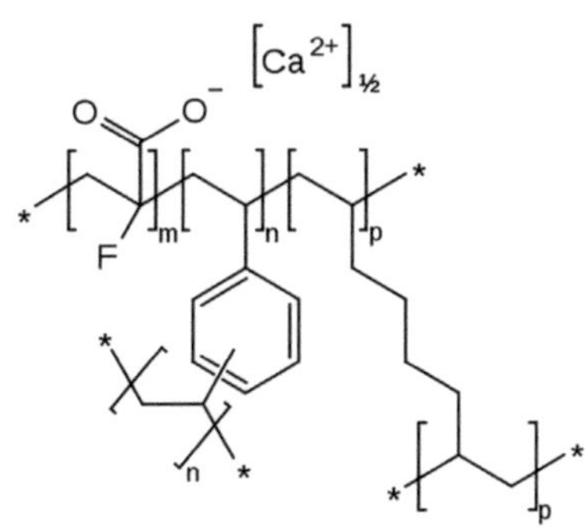

Figure 2.
Chemical structure of patiromer. (by Anypodetos – Own work, based on RxList, CC0, https://commons.wikimedia.org/w/index.php?curid=45569546).

5.1.1 Clinical pharmacology

Patiromer, which is sold under the brand name *Veltassa*, is a cation exchange polymer that binds potassium in the colon in exchange for calcium. The net result is increased fecal excretion of potassium with subsequent reduction in the serum potassium level. It is available as a powder for oral suspension that is taken once daily without regard to food. The initial dose is 8.4 grams, and if needed, the dose can be increased after a week to 16.8 grams to a maximum of 25.2 grams once daily [33, 41, 42].

It is a slowly–acting drug with an onset of action of 7 hours after administration, and the potassium level continues to decrease for at least 48 hours if treatment is continued [42]. The potassium level remains stable for 24 hours after administration of the last dose and does not increase before the next dose [42]. If patiromer is discontinued, the potassium level starts to rise again at least four days from the last dose [42]. Patiromer is not absorbed from the gut, is not metabolized, and is excreted unchanged with feces [41, 42].

5.1.2 Indication and utilization

Patiromer is indicated for the management of chronic hyperkalemia, especially for those who are on RAASi therapy [38–40]. Because patiromer acts relatively slowly, it is not usually recommended as an emergency treatment for life-threatening hyperkalemia. However, some data suggest that patiromer can acutely reduce serum potassium within 2 hours in patients with severe hyperkalemia [43]. Therefore, different guidelines are now recommending using patiromer in acute settings for patients with severe hyperkalemia alongside the standard of care [26, 37, 44].

5.1.3 Available evidence

- DIAMOND trial (Butler et al. – 2022): A multicenter, randomized, double-blind, placebo-controlled study on the use of patiromer in patients with hyperkalemia on RAASi therapy and/or on mineralocorticoid receptor antagonists (MRA). It included 878 patients with heart failure with reduced ejection fraction with a follow-up period of up to 43 weeks (median 27 weeks). Almost 42.4% of patients had stage 3 CKD. Patiromer significantly reduced the serum potassium level and reduced the MRA discontinuation or dose reduction [45].

- AMBER trial (Agarwal et al. – 2018): A multicenter, randomized, double-blind, placebo-controlled study on the use of patiromer in patients with CKD and resistant hypertension requiring spironolactone. It included 295 patients with a follow-up period of up to 12 weeks. It concluded that patiromer enabled more patients to continue treatment with spironolactone with less hyperkalemia [46].

- TOURMALINE trial (Pergola et al. – 2017): An open-label-randomized study on the efficacy and safety of patiromer administered once daily with or without food. It included 114 adult patients with hyperkalemia, of which 75.9% had CKD. It concluded that patiromer is equally effective and well tolerated when taken without food or with food, thereby offering the potential for dosing flexibility [47].

- OPAL-HK trial (Weir et al. – 2015): A multinational, randomized, single-blind, and placebo-controlled study on CKD patients receiving RAASi therapy who had hyperkalemia. It included 243 with a follow-up period of 12 weeks. It concluded that patiromer treatment was associated with a decrease in serum potassium levels and, as compared with placebo, a reduction in the recurrence of hyperkalemia [48].

- AMETHYST-DN trial (Bakris et al. – 2015): A multicenter, randomized, open-label study evaluating the efficacy and safety of patiromer in hyperkalemic patients with type 2 diabetes and CKD. It included 306 patients with a follow-up period of 52 weeks. It concluded that patiromer resulted in statistically significant decreases in serum potassium levels after 4 weeks of treatment, lasting through 52 weeks [49].

- PEARL-HF Study (Pitt et al. – 2011): A randomized, double-blind, placebo-controlled study evaluating the efficacy of patiromer on serum potassium levels and safety in patients with chronic heart failure receiving the standard therapy (with or without CKD) and spironolactone. It included 105 patients with a follow-up period of 4 weeks. It concluded that patiromer significantly reduced potassium levels and is well tolerated in patients with HF receiving standard therapy and spironolactone [50].

5.1.4 Side effects of patiromer

Patiromer is generally well tolerated [42]. Its safety and tolerability in clinical practice are predictable and consistent with clinical trial data [50].

Reported side effects were uncommon and mild, and did not lead to stopping patiromer [42, 51]. These include:

- Gastrointestinal side effects: constipation (6.9–7.2%), diarrhea (3.5–4.8%), abdominal discomfort (1.4–2%), flatulence (1.3–2%), nausea (1.7–2.3%). These side effects are usually mild and do not appear to be dose-dependent. In most cases, they improve spontaneously. The currently available evidence indicates that patiromer does not cause severe gastrointestinal complications, such as gastrointestinal ischemia, necrosis, or perforation.

- Electrolyte disturbance: Hypokalemia of less than 3.5 mmol/L may occur in 4.7–5% of patients. Mild to moderate hypomagnesemia may also occur with a risk ranging between 0.02–5.3%. Therefore, serum magnesium level should be monitored for at least 1 month after initiating patiromer. Because patiromer exchanges calcium for potassium, there is a theoretical risk of hypercalcemia, however, this risk is very uncommon and may occur in 0.06 and 0.09% of patients.

- Hypersensitivity reactions may occur in 0.3% of patients.

- Mild hypotension has been reported in 8% of patients.

- Drug interaction: patiromer can bind with other drugs in the gastrointestinal tract and decrease their absorption. The most clinically important interactions are with ciprofloxacin, thyroxine, and metformin. Therefore, these drugs should be administered more than three hours before or after patiromer [52].

Serious events like requirement of dialysis, sudden death, myocardial infarction, and sudden cardiac death were not seen in the global pharmacovigilance database [51].

5.2 Sodium zirconium cyclosilicate (SZC)

SZC has a unique crystal lattice structure, and its chemical formula is Na ~ 1.5H ~ 0.5ZrSi3O92–3H2O. See **Figure 3** [54].

5.2.1 Clinical pharmacology

Sodium zirconium cyclosilicate (SZC), which is sold under the brand name *Lokelma*, is an inorganic, insoluble compound that binds potassium in the colon in exchange for hydrogen and sodium. Binding of potassium reduces the concentration of free potassium in the gastrointestinal lumen, which leads to increased fecal excretion of potassium and lowering of serum potassium level.

SZC is available as a powder for oral suspension, and its starting or loading dose is 10 grams three times a day for 48 hours, followed by a maintenance dose of 5 grams daily. The dose could then be gradually increased, if needed, at a weekly interval to a maximum of 15 grams per day [54].

SZC has an onset of action of 1 hour, i.e., reduction in serum potassium level is observed one hour after initiation of therapy. However, serum potassium concentrations continue to decline over the 48-hour of the loading dose. Patients with higher starting serum potassium levels or receiving a higher dose have greater reductions in serum potassium level [54]. SZC is not systemically absorbed, it is not metabolized, and it is excreted unchanged with feces [54].

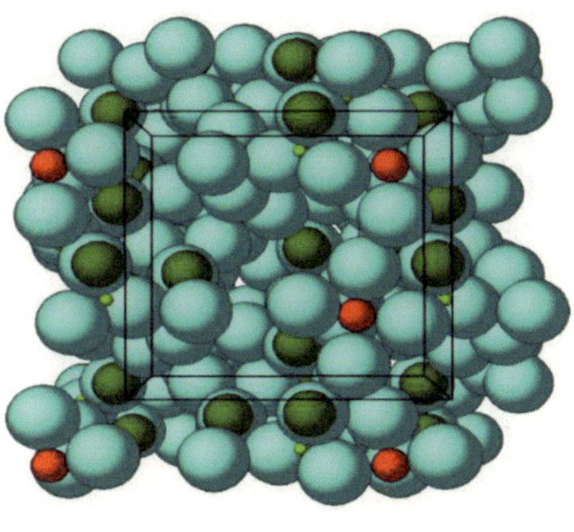

Figure 3.
Crystal structure of sodium zirconium cyclosilicate. Blue spheres = oxygen atoms, red spheres = zirconium atoms, green spheres = silicon atoms. (Ref. [53], https://commons.wikimedia.org/w/index.php?curid=44596225).

5.2.2 Indication and utilization

SZC is indicated for the management of chronic hyperkalemia, especially in patients receiving RAASi therapy [54]. As with patiromer, SZC was not initially approved in acute setting for the management of life-threatening hyperkalemia. But again, as with patiromer, data suggest that SCZ can acutely reduce potassium levels [55]. Therefore, different guidelines including the National Institute for Health and Care Excellence have recommended the use of SCZ for acute life-threatening hyperkalemia, in conjunction with standard care [26, 56]. In fact, for acute management of hyperkalemia, SZC is preferred over patiromer because of its more rapid onset of action [37].

5.2.3 Available evidence

- HARMONIZE-GLOBAL trial (Zannad et al. - 2020): A multi-center, randomized, double-blind, placebo-controlled studying the effect of SZC on outpatients with hyperkalemia (76.4% were on RAASi,78.3% had CKD). It included 267 patients with a follow-up period of 28 days. It concluded that SZC is more effective than placebo in achieving normokalemia at 48 hours; and can maintain it up to 28 days [57].

- HARMONIZE OLE trial (Roger et al. - 2019): An open-label extension (OLE) of the HARMONIZE study evaluating the efficacy and safety of SZC for ≤11 months in outpatients with serum K+ level 3.5–6.2 mmol/L. It included 123 patients (68.6% were on RAASi, 74% had eGFR <60 ml/minute/1.73 m2) with a follow-up period of ≤337 days. It found that SZC was able to achieve the target potassium level for ≤11 months during ongoing SZC treatment [58].

- ZS-005 trial (Spinowitz et al. - 2019): A multi-center, open-label study evaluating the use of SZC on adult outpatients with hyperkalemia (65% were on RAASi, 74% had eGFR <60 ml/minute/1.73 m**2**). It included 751 patients with a 52-week follow-up period. It concluded that SZC was associated with maintenance of normokalemia without substantial changes in RAASi therapy for ≤12 months [59].

- ZS-003 trial (Packham et al. - 2015): A multi-center, randomized, double-blind, placebo-controlled study evaluating the use of SCZ for the management of adult outpatients with hyperkalemia (66.7% were on RAASi, 74.5% had an eGFR <60 ml/minute/1.73 m**2**). It included 754 patients with a follow-up period of 16 days. It concluded that patients with hyperkalemia who received SZC, as compared with those who received placebo, had a significant reduction in potassium levels at 48 hours, with normokalemia maintained during 12 days of maintenance therapy [60].

- HARMONIZE trial (Kosiborod et al. - 2014): A multi-center, randomized, double-blind, placebo-controlled study evaluating the efficacy and safety of SZC for adult outpatients with hyperkalemia (69.8% on RAASi, 66% had an eGFR <60 ml/minute/1.73 m^2). It included 258 patients with a follow-up period of 28 days. It concluded that SZC is more effective than placebo in achieving normokalemia at 48 hours and maintaining it for 28 days [61].

5.2.4 Side effects of SZC

SZC is generally well tolerated, and there were no reported serious adverse events in clinical trials involving SZC [54, 58]. Reported side effects were [54, 57]:

- Hypokalemia: in clinical trials, hypokalemia (defined as serum potassium less than 3.5 mmol/L) developed in 4.1% of treated patients. Hypokalemia resolved with dose adjustment or discontinuation of SZC.

- Edema-related events ((edema, generalized edema, and peripheral edema): SZC contains approximately 400 mg sodium per 5 g dose. In placebo-controlled trials in which patients were treated with once-daily doses of SZC for up to 28 days, edema was reported in 4.4% of patients receiving 5 g, 5.9% of patients receiving 10 g, and 16.1% of patients receiving 15 g SZC compared to 2.4% of patients receiving placebo. In longer-term uncontrolled trials in which most patients were maintained on doses s < 15 g once daily, edema was reported in 8–11% of patients. Edema was generally mild to moderate in severity [54]. Patients need to be instructed to reduce their salt intake, and adjusting the diuretic dose may be required.

When using SZC, the following precautions must be considered [54]:

- Drug-interaction: SZC may transiently increase gastric pH and can change the absorption of co-administered drugs that exhibit pH-dependent solubility (e.g., furosemide, atorvastatin, and dabigatran), potentially leading to altered efficacy or safety of these drugs. Therefore, other oral medications should be administered at least 2 hours before or 2 hours after SZC.

- SZC safety and efficacy were not studied in patients with severe constipation or impaction, bowel obstruction, postoperative patients, or patients with bowel motility disorders; so it may be ineffective or may worsen these conditions. Therefore, it must be avoided in such patients.

- SZC agent has radio-opaque properties and, therefore, may appear when imaging the abdomen with X-ray of computed scans. This is to be considered in patients receiving SZC to avoid improper analysis of imaging [62].

Considering all aforementioned data showing the efficacy of patiromer and SCZ in reducing the potassium level, nephrologists are now able to use these novel binders to control chronic hyperkalemia in patients with CKD. Moreover, these binders will facilitate the optimization of RAASi therapy in such patients. RAASi medications are disease-modifying therapies in patients with CKD, and before the era of these novel binders, nephrologists would either reduce the dose or discontinue RAASi therapy in response to their common side effect of hyperkalemia. Now that patiromer and SCZ are mitigating this risk, they are functioning as "RAASi enablers" and allowing for RAASi proper utilization and dose optimization. Such an "enabling" effect was seen mainly as a secondary outcome in the previously summarized randomized studies of each binder. However, it was reproduced as a primary outcome of a meta-analysis of some of these studies [63]. This meta-analysis and systematic review investigated the efficacy of patiromer and SCZ on the optimization of RAASi therapy and reduction of hyperkalemia events [63]. Although the aim was to clarify the importance of their use in the clinical practice for heart failure patients, 2 of the 6 included studies targeted only CKD patients, and the remaining included a significant percentage of CKD patients [63]. This "enabling" effect may in the future extend the use of RAASi medications to other patients who are otherwise unable to take them due to hyperkalemia. The additional role of patiromer and SZC in managing acute hyperkalemia, together with the above-mentioned benefits, may reduce the risk of hospitalizations caused by hyperkalemia. This will reduce the economic burden and offset any cost associated with the acquisition of these drugs. **Table 2** mentions the cost of the available potassium binders. Based on cost-effective analyses, both patiromer and SCZ were cost-effective when used in patients with CKD [64, 65]. These novel potassium binders are changing the path of the management of CKD patients. Trials to evaluate whether these clinical practice benefits of patiromer and AZC result in a lower rate of major adverse events (e.g., mortality, requirement of dialysis, cardiac events...etc.) are still needed.

5.3 Novel potassium binders for dialysis patients

Patiromer is also effective in the management of pre-dialysis hyperkalemia in chronic hemodialysis patients [66, 67]. Because patiromer is not systemically absorbed, no dosage adjustment is necessary for any degree of kidney dysfunction [68]. Patiromer is unlikely to be dialyzed and no supplemental dose or dose adjustment necessary for hemodialysis, peritoneal dialysis or patients on prolonged or continuous renal replacement therapy [68].

SCZ can also be used for patients receiving chronic hemodialysis and have persistent pre-dialysis hyperkalemia [54, 69]. It is to be administered only on non-dialysis days, and the recommended starting dose is 5 grams once daily. If the pre-dialysis serum potassium is more than 6.5 mmol/L, SZC can be started at 10 grams once daily on non-dialysis [54]. Patients on chronic hemodialysis who are receiving SZC may develop significant hypokalemia and serum potassium levels must be closely monitored. During initiation and after a dose adjustment, assess serum potassium after one week [54]. SCZ is not systemically absorbed (or minimal absorption), so no dosage adjustment is necessary for patients with CKD or peritoneal dialysis patients [54].

6. Conclusions

The introduction of the novel potassium binders has filled a gap in the management of chronic hyperkalemia. Both patiromer and SZC have demonstrated their efficacy in maintaining normokalemia over the long term, in addition to their role in the short-term management of severe hyperkalemia [38]. This is particularly true for CKD patients, and more importantly, the fact that these novel binders enabled the continuation of RAASi therapy at stable or increased doses in many eligible patients (e.g., diabetes, CKD, heart failure patients) [38]. Patiromer and SZC are both generally well tolerated [38, 42, 51, 54, 58]. Common side effects of patiromer include hypomagnesemia, constipation, diarrhea, abdominal pain, and flatulence [42, 51]. Side effects of SZC treatment include constipation and edema-related events [54, 58]. For short and long-term management of hyperkalemia, it is encouraged to perform randomized controlled trials with a head-to-head comparison of efficacy and safety between patiromer and SZC. Additionally, trials to evaluate the effect of these novel potassium binders on clinical outcomes (e.g., mortalities, requirement of dialysis, cardiac events...etc) are required.

Acknowledgements

We would like to acknowledge the copyrights of **Figures 2** and **3** as indicated in the links posted below the figures.

Conflict of interest

The authors declare no conflict of interest.

Author details

Randah Dahlan* and Ali Alkatheeri
King Abdullah Medical City, Makkah, Saudi Arabia

*Address all correspondence to: randahdahlan@gmail.com

References

[1] Zacchia M, Abategiovanni ML, Stratigis S, Capasso G. Potassium: From physiology to clinical implications. Kidney Disease (Basel). 2016;**2**(2):72-79

[2] Stone MS, Martyn L, Weaver CM. Potassium intake, bioavailability, hypertension, and glucose control. Nutrients. 2016;**8**(7):444

[3] Watanabe R. Hyperkalemia in chronic kidney disease. Revista da Associação Médica Brasileira. 1992;**2020** (66Suppl. 1 (Suppl. 1)):s31-s36

[4] Mu F, Betts KA, Woolley JM, Dua A, Wang Y, Zhong J, et al. Prevalence and economic burden of hyperkalemia in the United States Medicare population. Current Medical Research and Opinion. 2020;**36**(8):1333-1341

[5] Palmer BF, Clegg DJ. Treatment of abnormalities of potassium homeostasis in CKD. Advances in Chronic Kidney Disease. 2017;**24**(5):319-324

[6] Belmar Vega L, Galabia ER, Bada da Silva J, Bentanachs González M, Fernández Fresnedo G, Piñera Haces C, et al. Epidemiology of hyperkalemia in chronic kidney disease. Nefrologia (Engl Ed). 2019;**39**(3):277-286

[7] Sarafidis PA, Blacklock R, Wood E, Rumjon A, Simmonds S, Fletcher-Rogers J, et al. Prevalence and factors associated with hyperkalemia in predialysis patients followed in a low-clearance clinic. Clinical Journal of the American Society of Nephrology. 2012;**7**(8):1234-1241

[8] Provenzano M, Minutolo R, Chiodini P, Bellizzi V, Nappi F, Russo D, et al. Competing-risk analysis of death and end stage kidney Disease by hyperkalaemia status in non-dialysis chronic kidney Disease patients receiving stable nephrology care. Journal of Clinical Medicine. 2018;**7**(12):499

[9] Luo J, Brunelli SM, Jensen DE, Yang A. Association between serum potassium and outcomes in patients with reduced kidney function. Clinical Journal of the American Society of Nephrology. 2016;**11**(1):90-100

[10] Thomsen RW, Nicolaisen SK, Hasvold P, Sanchez RG, Pedersen L, Adelborg K, et al. Elevated potassium levels in patients with chronic kidney disease: Occurrence, risk factors and clinical outcomes-a Danish population-based cohort study. Nephrology, Dialysis, Transplantation. 2018;**33**(9):1610-1620

[11] Hunter RW, Bailey MA. Hyperkalemia: Pathophysiology, risk factors and consequences. Nephrology, Dialysis, Transplantation. 2019;**34** (Suppl. 3):iii2-iii11

[12] Kovesdy CP, Matsushita K, Sang Y, Brunskill NJ, Carrero JJ, Chodick G, et al. CKD prognosis consortium. Serum potassium and adverse outcomes across the range of kidney function: A CKD prognosis consortium meta-analysis. European Heart Journal. 2018;**39**(17):1535-1542

[13] Horne L, Ashfaq A, MacLachlan S, Sinsakul M, Qin L, LoCasale R, et al. Epidemiology and health outcomes associated with hyperkalemia in a primary care setting in England. BMC Nephrology. 2019;**20**(1):85

[14] Rossignol P, Ruilope LM, Cupisti A, Ketteler M, Wheeler DC, Pignot M, et al. Recurrent hyperkalaemia management and use of renin-angiotensin-aldosterone

system inhibitors: A European multinational targeted chart review. Clinical Kidney Journal. 2019;**13**(4):714-719

[15] Brenner BM, Cooper ME, de Zeeuw D, Keane WF, Mitch WE, Parving HH, et al. RENAAL study Investigators. Effects of losartan on renal and cardiovascular outcomes in patients with type 2 diabetes and nephropathy. The New England Journal of Medicine. 2001;**345**(12):861-869

[16] Remuzzi G, Benigni A, Remuzzi A. Mechanisms of progression and regression of renal lesions of chronic nephropathies and diabetes. The Journal of Clinical Investigation. 2006;**116**(2):288-296

[17] Xie X, Liu Y, Perkovic V, Li X, Ninomiya T, Hou W, et al. Renin-angiotensin system inhibitors and kidney and cardiovascular outcomes in patients with CKD: A Bayesian network meta-analysis of randomized clinical trials. American Journal of Kidney Diseases. 2016;**67**(5):728-741

[18] Cheung AK, Chang TI, Cushman WC, Furth SL, Hou FF, Ix JH, et al. Executive summary of the KDIGO 2021 clinical practice guideline for the Management of Blood Pressure in chronic kidney Disease. Kidney International. 2021;**99**(3):559-569

[19] Lewis EJ, Hunsicker LG, Clarke WR, Berl T, Pohl MA, Lewis JB, et al. Collaborative study group. Renoprotective effect of the angiotensin-receptor antagonist irbesartan in patients with nephropathy due to type 2 diabetes. The New England Journal of Medicine. 2001;**345**(12):851-860

[20] Epstein M, Reaven NL, Funk SE, McGaughey KJ, Oestreicher N, Knispel J. Evaluation of the treatment gap between clinical guidelines and the utilization of renin-angiotensin-aldosterone system inhibitors. The American Journal of Managed Care. 2015;**21**(11 Suppl):S212-S220

[21] Yildirim T, Arici M, Piskinpasa S, Aybal-Kutlugun A, Yilmaz R, Altun B, et al. Major barriers against renin-angiotensin-aldosterone system blocker use in chronic kidney disease stages 3-5 in clinical practice: A safety concern? Renal Failure. 2012;**34**(9):1095-1099

[22] Linde C, Bakhai A, Furuland H, Evans M, McEwan P, Ayoubkhani D, et al. Real-world associations of renin-angiotensin-aldosterone system inhibitor dose, Hyperkalemia, and adverse clinical outcomes in a cohort of patients with new-onset chronic kidney Disease or heart failure in the United Kingdom. Journal of the American Heart Association. 2019;**8**(22):e012655. DOI: 10.1161/JAHA.119.012655 Epub 2019 Nov 12. Erratum in: J Am Heart Assoc. 2019 Dec 3;8(23): e014500

[23] Krishnan AV, Phoon RK, Pussell BA, Charlesworth JA, Bostock H, Kiernan MC. Altered motor nerve excitability in end-stage kidney disease. Brain. 2005;**128**(Pt 9): 2164-2174

[24] Arnold R, Pianta TJ, Pussell BA, Kirby A, O'Brien K, Sullivan K, et al. Randomized, controlled trial of the effect of dietary potassium restriction on nerve function in CKD. Clinical Journal of the American Society of Nephrology. 2017;**12**(10):1569-1577

[25] Zhang J, He X, Wu J. The impact of Hyperkalemia on mortality and healthcare resource utilization among patients with chronic kidney Disease: A matched cohort study in China. Frontiers in Public Health. 2022;**10**:855395

[26] Clase CM, Carrero JJ, Ellison DH, Grams ME, Hemmelgarn BR, Jardine MJ, et al. Conference participants. Potassium homeostasis and management of dyskalemia in kidney diseases: Conclusions from a kidney Disease: Improving global outcomes (KDIGO) controversies conference. Kidney International. 2020;**97**(1):42-61

[27] Costa D, Patella G, Provenzano M, Ielapi N, Faga T, Zicarelli M, et al. Hyperkalemia in CKD: An overview of available therapeutic strategies. Frontiers in Medicine (Lausanne). 2023;**10**:1178140

[28] Disease K. Improving global outcomes (KDIGO) CKD work group KDIGO 2012 clinical practice guideline for the evaluation and management of chronic kidney disease. Kidney International. Supplement. 2013;**3**:1-150

[29] Palmer BF, Colbert G, Clegg DJ. Potassium homeostasis, chronic kidney Disease, and the plant-enriched diets. Kidney360. 2020;**1**(1):65-71

[30] Parks M, Grady D. Sodium Polystyrene Sulfonate for Hyperkalemia. JAMA Internal Medicine. 2019;**179**(8):1023-1024

[31] Tinawi M. Potassium Binders. Archives of Internal Medicine Research. 2020;**3**:141-145

[32] Lepage L, Dufour AC, Doiron J, Handfield K, Desforges K, Bell R, et al. Randomized clinical trial of sodium polystyrene sulfonate for the treatment of mild Hyperkalemia in CKD. Clinical Journal of the American Society of Nephrology. 2015;**10**(12):2136-2142

[33] Food and Drug Administration Safety. Kayexelate: Sodium Polystyrene Sulfonate, USP, Cation-Exchange Resin. Available from: https://www.accessdata.fda.gov/drugsatfda_docs/label/2009/011287s022lbl.pdf

[34] Harel Z, Harel S, Shah PS, Wald R, Perl J, Bell CM. Gastrointestinal adverse events with sodium polystyrene sulfonate (Kayexalate) use: A systematic review. The American Journal of Medicine. 2013;**126**(3):264.e9-264.24

[35] Laureati P, Xu Y, Trevisan M, Schalin L, Mariani I, Bellocco R, et al. Initiation of sodium polystyrene sulphonate and the risk of gastrointestinal adverse events in advanced chronic kidney disease: A nationwide study. Nephrology, Dialysis, Transplantation. 2020;**35**(9):1518-1526

[36] Noel JA, Bota SE, Petrcich W, Garg AX, Carrero JJ, Harel Z, et al. Risk of hospitalization for serious adverse gastrointestinal events associated with sodium polystyrene sulfonate use in patients of advanced age. JAMA Internal Medicine. 2019;**179**(8):1025-1033

[37] Mount D. Treatment and prevention of hyperkalemia in adults. In: Sterns R, editor. UpToDate. Waltham, MA: UpToDate; 2023. [Accessed: 30 December 2023]

[38] De Nicola L, Ferraro PM, Montagnani A, Pontremoli R, Dentali F, Sesti G. Recommendations for the management of hyperkalemia in patients receiving renin-angiotensin-aldosterone system inhibitors. Internal and Emergency Medicine. 2024;**19**(2):295-306

[39] Disease K. Improving global outcomes (KDIGO) diabetes work group. KDIGO 2020 clinical practice guideline for diabetes Management in Chronic Kidney Disease. Kidney International. 2020;**98**(4S):S1-S115

[40] Disease K. Improving global outcomes (KDIGO) blood pressure work group. KDIGO 2021 clinical practice guideline for the Management of Blood

Pressure in chronic kidney Disease. Kidney International. 2021;**99**(3S):S1-S87

[41] Esposito P, Conti NE, Falqui V, Cipriani L, Picciotto D, Costigliolo F, et al. New treatment options for Hyperkalemia in patients with chronic kidney Disease. Journal of Clinical Medicine. 2020;**9**(8):2337

[42] Bushinsky DA, Williams GH, Pitt B, Weir MR, Freeman MW, Garza D, et al. Patiromer induces rapid and sustained potassium lowering in patients with chronic kidney disease and hyperkalemia. Kidney International. 2015;**88**(6):1427-1433

[43] Rafique Z, Liu M, Staggers KA, Minard CG, Peacock WF. Patiromer for treatment of Hyperkalemia in the emergency department: A pilot study. Academic Emergency Medicine. 2020;**27**(1):54-60

[44] National Institute for Health and Care Excellence. Patiromer for Treating Hyperkalemia. National Institute for Health and Care Excellence website. Available from: https://www.nice.org.uk/guidance/ta623/chapter/1-Recommendations. Accessed January 3, 2024

[45] Butler J, Anker SD, Lund LH, Coats AJS, Filippatos G, Siddiqi TJ, et al. Patiromer for the management of hyperkalemia in heart failure with reduced ejection fraction: The DIAMOND trial. European Heart Journal. 2022;**43**(41):4362-4373

[46] Agarwal R, Rossignol P, Romero A, Garza D, Mayo MR, Warren S, et al. Patiromer versus placebo to enable spironolactone use in patients with resistant hypertension and chronic kidney disease (AMBER): A phase 2, randomized, double-blind, placebo-controlled trial. Lancet. 2019;**394**(10208):1540-1550

[47] Pergola PE, Spiegel DM, Warren S, Yuan J, Weir MR. Patiromer lowers serum potassium when taken without food: Comparison to dosing with food from an open-label, randomized, parallel group Hyperkalemia study. American Journal of Nephrology. 2017;**46**(4):323-332

[48] Weir MR, Bakris GL, Bushinsky DA, Mayo MR, Garza D, Stasiv Y, et al. OPAL-HK Investigators. Patiromer in patients with kidney disease and hyperkalemia receiving RAAS inhibitors. The New England Journal of Medicine. 2015;**372**(3):211-221

[49] Bakris GL, Pitt B, Weir MR, Freeman MW, Mayo MR, Garza D. Et al; AMETHYST-DN Investigators. Effect of Patiromer on serum potassium level in patients with Hyperkalemia and diabetic kidney Disease: The AMETHYST-DN randomized clinical trial. Journal of the American Medical Association. 2015;**314**(2):151-161

[50] Pitt B, Anker SD, Bushinsky DA, Kitzman DW, Zannad F, Huang IZ, et al. Evaluation of the efficacy and safety of RLY5016, a polymeric potassium binder, in a double-blind, placebo-controlled study in patients with chronic heart failure (the PEARL-HF) trial. European Heart Journal. 2011;**32**(7):820-828

[51] Rossignol P, David L, Chan C, Conrad A, Weir MR. Safety and tolerability of the potassium binder Patiromer from a global pharmacovigilance database collected over 4 years compared with data from the clinical trial program. Drugs Real World Outcomes. 2021;**8**(3):315-323

[52] Lesko LJ, Offman E, Brew CT, Garza D, Benton W, Mayo MR, et al. Evaluation of the potential for drug interactions with Patiromer in healthy volunteers. Journal of Cardiovascular Pharmacology and Therapeutics. 2017;**22**(5):434-446

[53] Stavros F, Yang A, Leon A, et al. Characterization of Structure and Function of ZS-9, a K+ Selective Ion Trap. PloS one. 2014;**9**(12):e114686. DOI: 10.1371/journal.pone.0114686

[54] Food and Drug Administration Safety: LOKELMA® (Sodium Zirconium Cyclosilicate) for Oral Suspension. Available from: https://www.accessdata.fda.gov/drugsatfda_docs/label/2018/207078s000lbl.pdf

[55] Peacock WF, Rafique Z, Vishnevskiy K, Michelson E, Vishneva E, Zvereva T, et al. Emergency potassium normalization treatment including sodium zirconium Cyclosilicate: A phase II, randomized, double-blind, placebo-controlled study (ENERGIZE). Academic Emergency Medicine. 2020;**27**(6):475-486

[56] National Institute for Health and Care Excellence. Sodium Zirconium Cyclosilicate for Treating Hyperkalemia: Guidance. National Institute for Health and Care Excellence website. Available from: https://www.nice.org.uk/guidance/ta599/chapter/1-Recommendations [Accessed January 3, 2024]

[57] Zannad F, Hsu BG, Maeda Y, Shin SK, Vishneva EM, Rensfeldt M, et al. Efficacy and safety of sodium zirconium cyclosilicate for hyperkalaemia: The randomized, placebo-controlled HARMONIZE-global study. ESC Heart Fail. 2020;7(1):54-64

[58] Roger SD, Spinowitz BS, Lerma EV, Singh B, Packham DK, Al-Shurbaji A, et al. Efficacy and safety of sodium zirconium Cyclosilicate for treatment of Hyperkalemia: An 11-month open-label extension of HARMONIZE. American Journal of Nephrology. 2019;**50**(6):473-480

[59] Spinowitz BS, Fishbane S, Pergola PE, Roger SD, Lerma EV, Butler J, et al. ZS-005 study Investigators. Sodium zirconium Cyclosilicate among individuals with Hyperkalemia: A 12-month phase 3 study. Clinical Journal of the American Society of Nephrology. 2019;**14**(6):798-809

[60] Packham DK, Rasmussen HS, Lavin PT, El-Shahawy MA, Roger SD, Block G, et al. Sodium zirconium cyclosilicate in hyperkalemia. The New England Journal of Medicine. 2015;**372**(3):222-231

[61] Kosiborod M, Rasmussen HS, Lavin P, Qunibi WY, Spinowitz B, Packham D, et al. Effect of sodium zirconium cyclosilicate on potassium lowering for 28 days among outpatients with hyperkalemia: The HARMONIZE randomized clinical trial. Journal of the American Medical Association. 2014;**312**(21):2223-2233

[62] Kolesnik M, Berezovsky D, Sayegh M, Samarneh M. Radiopacity of sodium zirconium cyclosilicate on CT imaging. CEN Case Reports. 2021;**10**(4):559-562

[63] Paolillo S, Basile C, Dell'Aversana S, Esposito I, Chirico A, Colella A, et al. Novel potassium binders to optimize RAASi therapy in heart failure: A systematic review and meta-analysis. European Journal of Internal Medicine. 2024;**119**:109-117

[64] Ward T, Lewis RD, Brown T, Baxter G, de Arellano AR. A cost-effectiveness analysis of patiromer in the UK: Evaluation of hyperkalaemia treatment and lifelong RAASi maintenance in chronic kidney disease patients with and without heart failure. BMC Nephrology. 2023;**24**(1):47

[65] Kim K, Fagerström J, Chen G, Lagunova Z, Furuland H, McEwan P. Cost effectiveness of sodium zirconium

cyclosilicate for the treatment of hyperkalemia in patients with CKD in Norway and Sweden. BMC Nephrology. 2022;**23**(1):281

[66] Amdur RL, Paul R, Barrows ED, Kincaid D, Muralidharan J, Nobakht E, et al. The potassium regulator patiromer affects serum and stool electrolytes in patients receiving hemodialysis. Kidney International. 2020;**98**(5):1331-1340

[67] Kovesdy CP, Rowan CG, Conrad A, Spiegel DM, Fogli J, Oestreicher N, et al. Real-world evaluation of Patiromer for the treatment of Hyperkalemia in Hemodialysis patients. Kidney International Reports. 2018;**4**(2):301-309

[68] Lexicomp. Patiromer: Drug Information. UpToDate. Waltham, MA: UpToDate; 2023 [Accessed: 4 January 2024]

[69] Fishbane S, Ford M, Fukagawa M, McCafferty K, Rastogi A, Spinowitz B, et al. A phase 3b, randomized, double-blind, placebo controlled study of sodium zirconium Cyclosilicate for reducing the incidence of Predialysis Hyperkalemia. Journal of the American Society of Nephrology. 2019;**30**(9):1723-1733